AF668219

Manual on

Practical Points in Treatment of Menopause

68th All India Congress of Obstetrics & Gynaecology

aicog Delhi 2026

Advocate Innovate Challenge Optimise Globalise

Manual on
Practical Points in Treatment of Menopause

Series Editors

Ashok Kumar
MD PhD
Director–Professor
Department of Obstetrics and Gynecology
Atal Bihari Vajpayee Institute of Medical Sciences
and Dr Ram Manohar Lohia Hospital
New Delhi, India

Madhavi M Gupta
MS
Director–Professor
Department of Obstetrics and Gynecology
Maulana Azad Medical College and Lok Nayak Hospital
New Delhi, India

K Aparna Sharma
MBBS MD
Professor
Department of Obstetrics and Gynecology
All India Institute of Medical Sciences
New Delhi, India

Editors

Manju Khemani
Maninder Ahuja
Archana Dwivedi
Shyjus P
Vinita Gupta

Co-Editors

Jyoti Bhaskar
Kiranjeet Kaur
Meenakshi Ahuja

JAYPEE BROTHERS MEDICAL PUBLISHERS
The Health Sciences Publisher
New Delhi | London

Message from Series Editors

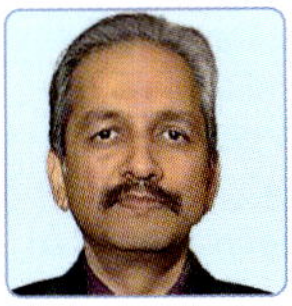

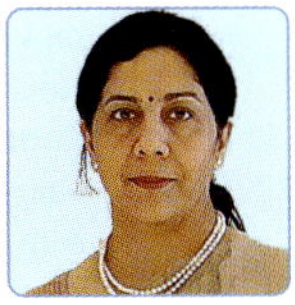

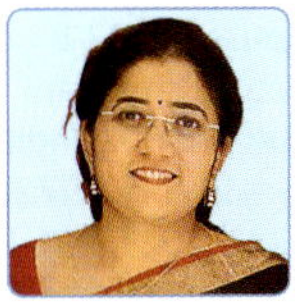

Ashok Kumar
Organizing Chairperson
AICOG-2026
New Delhi

Madhavi M Gupta
Organizing Secretary
AICOG-2026
New Delhi

K Aparna Sharma
Organizing Secretary
AICOG-2026
New Delhi

It is after 18 long years that the 68th AICOG is being held in New Delhi. It is a pleasure to welcome you all.

The Organizing Team have poured their heart and soul into curating an academic program which one will feel a loss if missed. The scientific sessions include both national and international faculty who are stalwarts in their fields. There are 18 workshops with 8 full-day and 5 each in the pre-lunch and post-lunch time.

On this occasion, the workshop faculty, have gone that extra mile to publish the workshop manual for eight workshops. This includes all recent scientific evidence and clinical management guidelines. These manuals will serve as a go-to evidence-based resource in your day-to-day clinical practice. We look forward to receiving your valuable feedback.

We acknowledge the hard work put in by all the editors, co-editors, and the authors, who, in spite of busy schedules and time constraints, have contributed immensely.

We would also like to thank M/s Jaypee Brothers Medical Publishers (P) Ltd, New Delhi, India, for partnering with us.

We sincerely hope that you will enjoy reading these manuals, find this manual useful, and treasure it for future use in your practical work.

We take this opportunity to wish you a memorable time during your stay in New Delhi.

Warm Regards

JAYPEE **Jaypee Brothers Medical Publishers (P) Ltd**

Headquarters
EMCA House, 23/23-B
Ansari Road, Daryaganj
New Delhi 110 002, India
Landline: +91-11-23272143, +91-11-23272703
+91-11-23282021, +91-11-23245672
e-mail: jaypee@jaypeebrothers.com

Corporate Office
4838/24, Ansari Road, Daryaganj
New Delhi 110 002, India
Phone: +91-11-43574357
Fax: +91-11-43574314
e-mail: jaypee@jaypeebrothers.com

Overseas Office
JP Medical Ltd.
83, Victoria Street, London
SW1H 0HW (UK)
Phone: +44-20 3170 8910
e-mail: info@jpmedpub.com

EU GPSR Authorised Representative
Logos Europe, 9 rue Nicolas Poussin
17000, La Rochelle, France
Phone: +33 (0) 6 67 93 73 78
e-mail: contact@logoseurope.eu

Website: www.jaypeebrothers.com
Website: www.jaypeedigital.com

Inquiries for bulk sales may be solicited at: jaypee@jaypeebrothers.com

Manual on Practical Points in Treatment of Menopause

First Edition: **2026**

ISBN: 978-93-7545-181-5

Printed at: Samrat Offset Pvt. Ltd.

Contributors

Aakansha Shukla MD
Resident
Department of Endocrinology
Sir Ganga Ram Hospital
New Delhi, India

Aarshika Singh MD FMAS DNB
Associate Consultant
Fortis La Femme
New Delhi, India

Ajay Aggarwal
MBBS DM (Endocrinology) MD (Medicine)
Chairperson, Endocrinologist
Department of Endocrinology
Sir Ganga Ram Hospital
New Delhi, India

Amrita Razdan Kaul MBBS DGO
Senior Consultant
Department of Obstetrics
and Gynecology Services
Asian Institute of Medical Sciences
Faridabad, Haryana, India

Anita Kant MBBS MD
Chairman and Head
Department of Obstetrics
and Gynecology Services
Asian Institute of Medical Sciences
Faridabad, Haryana, India

Archana Dwivedi
MBBS MB DGO FICOG CIMP FIMS
Director and Head
Department of Obstetrics
and Gynecology
Sterling Hospitals, Racecourse
Vadodara, Gujarat, India
Chairperson, FOGSI MMC

Binal Shah
MBBS MD Diploma Gynec Endoscopy
(Germany) FICOG CIMP
Consultant, Gynecologist
and Laparoscopic Surgeon
Dwarkesh Hospital
Vadodara, Gujarat, India

Bipasa Sen DGO DNB (Gynae)
Gynecologist
Department of Obstetrics
and Gynecology
Sterling Hospital
Kolkata, West Bengal, India

Jyoti Bhaskar MD FRCOG FICOG FICMCH
Additional Director
Cloudnine Hospital
New Delhi, India
Secretary, Delhi Menopause Society

Jyoti Jaiswal MBBS MD FICOG
Professor and Head
Department of Obstetrics
and Gynecology
Pt JNM Medical College
Raipur, Chhattisgarh, India

Kiran Aggarwal MD FICOG CIMP
Director Professor
Department of Obstetrics
and Gynecology
Lady Hardinge Medical College and
Smt Sucheta Kriplani Hospital
New Delhi, India

Kiranjeet Kaur
MBBS DGO DNB (Obs & Gyne)
Associate Director
Department of Obstetrics
and Gynecology
Cloudnine Hospital, New Delhi, India

Maninder Ahuja
MBBS DGO CIMP FICOG FIAOG
Senior Gynecologist
Ahuja Hospital and Infertility Centre
Faridabad, Haryana, India

Manju Varma MBBS MD
Former Professor and Head
Department of Obstetrics
and Gynecology, MLN Medical College
Prayagraj, Uttar Pradesh, India
President, Uttar Pradesh Chapter 2012
and 2013

Mayank Vashishtha
Department of Endocrinology
Sir Ganga Ram Hospital
New Delhi, India

Meenakshi Ahuja MD FICOG CIMP
Senior Director
Fortis La Femme
New Delhi, India
Chairperson, Website Committee
Indian Menopause Society

Neelam Aggarwal MBBS MD
Professor
Department of Obstetrics
and Gynecology
Maharishi Markandeshwar College
of Medical Science and Research
Ambala, Haryana, India

Renu Meena

Renuka Malik MBBS MD
Principal Consultant
(Obstetrics and Gynecology)
Atal Bihari Vajpayee Institute of
Medical Sciences and Dr RML Hospital
New Delhi, India
President, Delhi Menopause Society

Ruchika Garg MBBS MD
Professor
Department of Obstetrics
and Gynecology
SN Medical College
Agra, Uttar Pradesh, India
Editor-in-Chief, Journal of Midlife Health

Saraswathi Kondapalli MBBS MS
Associate Consultant
Department of Obstetrics and
Gynecology
Sterling Hospitals
Vadodara, Gujarat, India

Setu Gupta MD DM
Associate Consultant
Department of Endocrinology
and Metabolism
Department of Endocrinology
Sir Ganga Ram Hospital
New Delhi, India

Shubhi Gupta
MBBS MD
Assistant Professor
Department of Obstetrics
and Gynecology
Maharishi Markandeshwar College
of Medical Science and Research
Ambala, Haryana, India

Shyjus P MBBS MS
Consultant Gynecologist
Birla Fertility and
ARMC IVF Centre
Kannur, Kerala, India

SS Doda MD FICR
Director and Consultant Radiologist
Dr Doda's Diagnostics
and Healthcare
New Delhi, India

Suneeta Mittal
MBBS MD FRCOG (ae) FICOG FAMS FICMCH
FIMSA FICLS
Senior Director and Head
Department of Obstetrics
and Gynecology
Fortis Memorial Research Institute
Gurugram, Haryana, India

Taruna Dua MBBS DNB
Senior Consultant and Unit Head
Department of Obstetrics
and Gynecology
Aakash Healthcare Super Speciality
Hospital
New Delhi, India

Uma Vaidyanathan MS DGO MBBS
Director
Department of Obstetrics
and Gynecology
Fortis Hospital
New Delhi, India

Ushma Maniar DGO CIMP FICOG
Founder
Devamrut Hospital and
Vadodara Menopause Clinic
Vadodara, Gujarat, India

Preface

According to the Indian Menopausal Society, there will be 401 million women above 45 years of age by the year 2026. The mean age of menopause in India is 5 years earlier than that of their western counterpart. It is 46–47.5 years. There is a lack of awareness regarding the symptoms of menopause in the majority of women. It is equally important to address the hesitation in prescribing menopausal hormone therapy (MHT) in health care.

This manual has been written as a guide and ready reckoner for healthcare professionals to use in their day-to-day practice.

The first part of this booklet addresses prescription writing, and the second part is all about osteoporosis.

Osteoporosis remains one of the most under-recognized yet consequential noncommunicable diseases affecting women worldwide. Often termed the "silent disease," it progresses insidiously until a fracture occurs—frequently marking the beginning of pain, disability, loss of independence, and increased mortality. Despite advances in diagnostics and therapeutics, osteoporosis continues to be diagnosed late and treated inadequately, particularly in women.

This manual has been conceived to address a crucial gap in osteoporosis care: the need to shift focus from *fracture-driven management to prevention, early identification, and holistic intervention*. Osteoporosis is not a disease that begins at menopause or old age; rather, it is a *life-course condition*, influenced by nutrition, physical activity, hormonal transitions, metabolic health, environmental factors, and sociocultural determinants from adolescence onward.

In clinical practice, missed opportunities are common—risk factors are overlooked, bone health is not discussed during reproductive or midlife consultations, and fractures are often treated without addressing the underlying bone disease. This manual aims to equip healthcare professionals with *practical, evidence-based guidance* to recognize risk early, stratify patients appropriately, and institute timely, individualized care.

Designed as a *hands-on reference*, the manual integrates current scientific understanding with real-world clinical application. It covers risk assessment, screening strategies, interpretation of bone mineral density, role of nutrition and exercise, pharmacological options, fracture prevention, and long-term follow-up. Special emphasis is placed on women's health, menopause, and the Indian and South-Asian context, where nutritional deficiencies, early menopause, and limited awareness further compound risk.

Equally important is the recognition that osteoporosis care cannot exist in isolation. Effective management requires a *multidisciplinary and patient-centred approach*, involving gynecologists, physicians, orthopedicians, endocrinologists, physiotherapists, nutritionists, and primary care providers. Empowering women with knowledge and involving them as active partners in their care is central to improving outcomes.

This manual is intended for clinicians at all levels—postgraduate students, practicing physicians, and healthcare professionals—who seek a structured yet flexible guide to osteoporosis care. It is hoped that this work will help *break the silence surrounding osteoporosis*, reduce preventable fractures, and contribute to healthier, stronger aging for women.

Editors: **Manju Khemani, Maninder Ahuja, Archana Dwivedi, Shyjus P, Vinita Gupta**

Co-Editors: **Jyoti Bhaskar, Kiranjeet Kaur, Meenakshi Ahuja**

Contents

SECTION 1: Prescription Writing

Section Editor: **Manju Khemani**

SECTION 2: Break the Silence—Not the Bones: A Life Course Management of Osteoporosis

Section Editor: **Maninder Ahuja**

SECTION 1

Prescription Writing

Section Editor: ***Manju Khemani***

1 CHAPTER

Overview of Menopause Hormone Therapy

Shyjus P

INTRODUCTION

Menopause is defined retrospectively when a woman has an amenorrhea of 12 months with loss of ovarian function for which no other pathology can be assigned.

Symptoms due to the lack of estrogen are vasomotor flushes, an increase in visceral fat, metabolic dysfunction, psychological upsets, vulvovaginal atrophy, sexual dysfunction etc.

These differ across populations, race, culture, ethnicity and also due to socioeconomic and personal factors like smoking etc.

The presentation also varies according to age and the time duration of menopause and associated comorbidities like obesity, hypertension, diabetes, etc.

The journey that we have made, with the use of hormones for women at or beyond menopause, is more than just interesting. From those days when it was considered as something that every menopausal woman need to use to remain feminine, to the present day where we have specific indications to use it, the journey has had its ups and downs. From being injudiciously prescribed for all women to an almost sudden stoppage due to the concerns raised by the WHI trial results, thankfully, now we are almost settling down to a recommended pattern for writing a menopausal prescription.

HISTORY

Diethylstilbestrol and conjugated equine estrogens (CEE) were the earlier estrogens used for treating vasomotor symptoms. It used to be estrogen-only therapy then, and soon came the realization about the risk of endometrial cancer. Adding progesterone was found to counter this risk.

Earlier studies indicated bone and heart benefits of estrogen, which led to the conduct of a large-scale randomized controlled prevention trial, the *Women's Health Initiative* (WHI). Women were randomized to receive either combined hormone therapy (HT), ET, or placebo, and the effects of therapy on coronary heart disease (CHD), stroke, venous thromboembolism, fractures, and cancers were to be observed over 10 years. However, in 2002, WHI had to be stopped early because evidence linked HT to a slightly increased risk of stroke, heart disease, and breast cancer.

There was a lot of hue and cry against MHT around the world as the WHI results became public. This led to the sudden and massive dip in the use of MHT across the world. It was only ten years later that a re-analysis of the WHI data revealed that the issue was with the age at which MHT was given in these women, which also brought in the window of opportunity hypothesis. The average age of women in the Women's Health Initiative (WHI) study was 63 years. Publications from the WHI reinforced the efficacy of the beneficial effects of estrogens on menopausal symptoms and bones. Further, cardioprotection was seen when MHT was started in healthy early postmenopausal women. Since then, more evidence has been gathered. The Danish Osteoporosis Prevention Study (DOPS) study and E3N studies proved the superiority of 17 beta-estradiol over conjugated equine estrogens. The better safety profile that the more natural progesterones, including micronized progesterone and dydrogesterone, can give, over the earlier used agents like medroxyprogesterone, has also been established.

CONCEPTS IN PRESCRIBING MHT

Hormone therapy at menopause would include prescribing estrogens, progestogens, combined E+P therapy, androgens and tibolone to the needy women. These are available in different formulations, combinations and with different potencies. Oral, transdermal, and vaginal preparations are the most commonly preferred routes.

- Multiple routes and multiple formulations provide the much-needed flexibility to MHT to suit the needs of the women. The risk-benefit ratio varies with the age of the woman, the number of years since menopause, presence of co-morbidities, the type of hormone used and the route.
- The indications for prescribing MHT are moderate to severe vasomotor symptoms and genitourinary syndrome of menopause.
- It is also used for the prevention and treatment of osteoporosis in some countries.
- MHT is safest when used before the age of 60 years or within 10 years of menopause.
- For women with symptoms limited to vaginal dryness or dyspareunia, estrogens applied locally at the vagina at the lowest dose is the recommended option.
- When vaginal estrogens are used, there is no need to even add progesterone, even in a woman with an intact uterus.
- The dose of MHT should be low to start with and stepped up as needed
- When used for the above-mentioned indications, MHT gives certain additional benefits in the form of better sleep, less muscle and joint

pains, lesser mood disorders, better sexual function and better quality of life, decrease in colon cancer risk, decrease in diabetes and metabolic syndrome and possible benefits in CVD and cognitive function

- MHT is an effective treatment for the prevention of fractures in at-risk women before the age of 60 years or within 10 years after menopause.
- Use of Androgenic preparations as part of MHT may improve both sexuality and overall quality of life.
- For women with premature ovarian insufficiency, experts recommend using systemic MHT at the standard dose till they reach the average age of natural menopause.

The option of MHT is an individual decision in terms of quality of life and health priorities, personal risk factors, and co-morbidities.

BEFORE PRESCRIBING MHT

Before prescribing MHT, consider the stage and duration of menopause, symptoms of menopause, and contraindications.

The woman needs to be fully informed of all the likely benefits, as well as the potential risks. She should have a full physical and gynecological examination with special emphasis on blood pressure, breasts, abdomen, and pelvic organs. Investigations including a complete blood count, HBA1C, Lipid profile and TSH can be looked at. Pap smear, USG examination of abdomen and pelvis and a Mammography are also preferably advised.

Which hormones?

The hormones commonly prescribed are estrogen, progestogen/progesterone and tibolone

Types of Estrogen:

- *Estradiol:* 17 beta-estradiol, estradiol hemihydrate, estradiol valerate
- Conjugated equine estrogen tablets for oral use containing several molecules of estrone, equine, and other estrogens. Each tablet contains 0.3 mg or 0.625 mg of conjugated estrogens.
- Estriol is available as a vaginal cream
- *Progesterones:* Dydrogesterone, micronized progesterone

Intrauterine Levonorgestrel System has been used with success as the progestogenic component of hormone therapy for menopausal symptoms

Tibolone is a synthetic steroid compound. This on absorption is converted in vivo to metabolites with estrogenic, progestogenic, and androgenic actions. It is used at a dose of 2.5 mg/day to treat vasomotor symptoms, mood disorders and reduced libido.

How is MHT given?

Estrogen alone therapy is used in women without a uterus. In all women with an intact uterus, progesterone needs to be added to the estrogen, while giving MHT.

Estradiol 1,2 mg or conjugated estrogens 0.625–1.25 mg daily is the usual starting dose for women without a uterus, where a continuous regimen is recommended.

When Estrogen and Progesterone need to be combined, it is either given continuously or sequentially. Sequential regime means adding progesterone for 10–14 days every month, along with estrogen, which is given on all days.

The dose of the continuous regime for estradiol and dydrogesterone are 0.5 mg/2.5 mg and 1 mg/5 mg, given every day without a break between packs. 1mg of estradiol and 100 mg of micronized progesterone is the other combination used for continuous regime. If a sequential regime is used , dose the dydrogesterone will be 10 mg and the dose of micronized progesterone will be 200 mg, given for 10–14 days every month.

In women experiencing natural menopause, treatment should commence no earlier than at least 12 months after their last natural menstrual bleed. For surgically-induced menopause, treatment may start immediately.

CONTRAINDICATIONS FOR MHT

- Active endometrial and gynecological hormone dependent cancers Active breast cancer and estrogen-progestogen receptor-positive cancers
- Known or suspected pregnancy
- Undiagnosed, abnormal vaginal bleeding
- Severe active liver disease with impaired/abnormal liver function
- Estrogen-dependent venous thrombosis
- Inherent increased risk of thromboembolism

RELATIVE CONTRAINDICATIONS

- Migraine headaches
- Superficial thrombophlebitis
- Strong family history of breast cancer
- Uterine fibroids
- Endometriosis
- Gallbladder disease
- Established CVD

CONCLUSION

With enough updated evidence available today about the safety, every OBGyn should be in a position to prescribe MHT for the needy woman. From being thought as a panacea for all, MHT is now given for specific indications, including moderate to severe vasomotor symptoms and for managing GUSM. It is best given to a woman under 60 years of age and within 10 years of menopause. With the availability of newer formulations including the transdermal gels and a better understanding of the dosages to be used, the safety profile of MHT can be extended, so that almost every needy women can safely receive it.

SUGGESTED READING

1. Eden J. The endometrial and breast safety of menopausal hormone therapy containing micronized progesterone: a short review. Aust N Z J Obstet Gynaecol. 2017;57(1):12-5.
2. Meeta M, Digumarti L, Agarwal N, et al. Clinical practice guidelines on menopause: an executive summary and recommendations: Indian Menopause Society 2019-2020. J Midlife Health. 2020;11(2):55-95.
3. Schierbeck LL, Rejnmark L, Tofteng CL, et al. Effect of hormone replacement therapy on cardiovascular events in recently postmenopausal women: a randomized trial. BMJ. 2012;345.
4. Stefanick M. Estrogens and progestins: background and history, trends use, and guidelines and regimens approved by the US Food and Drug Administration. Am J Med. 2005;118(12B):64-73.
5. Women's Health Initiative Study Group. Design of the women's health initiative clinical trial and observational study. Control Clin Trials. 1998;19(1):61-109.

2 CHAPTER

Evaluation of Indications and Patients of MHT

Jyoti Bhaskar

INTRODUCTION

The use of Menopause Hormone Therapy (MHT), previously known as Hormone Replacement Therapy (HRT), has been one of the most debated subjects in women's health over the past three decades. The pendulum of opinion has swung from widespread use in the 1980s and 1990s to a significant decline after the initial results of the Women's Health Initiative (WHI) study in 2002, which linked hormone therapy with potential cardiovascular and cancer risks. However, reanalysis of data and subsequent trials have demonstrated that the risks and benefits of MHT depend heavily on the age of initiation, timing of therapy, type of hormone, route of administration, and individual patient profile.

Today, the focus has shifted toward individualized, evidence-based therapy to optimize benefits while minimizing risks.

EVALUATION OF A WOMAN BEFORE STARTING MHT

Right Indication

Clearly define the Indication for starting MHT.

Core Indications of MHT

Vasomotor Symptoms (VMS)

Hot flushes and night sweats are among the most distressing symptoms of menopause, affecting up to 75% of women. VMS may start during the menopause transition, reach maximum intensity during the first 2 years postmenopause, and then decline over the next 6 months to 2 years. However, some may experience it for 10 years or longer. Estrogen therapy remains the most effective treatment, reducing frequency and severity by up to 80–90%.

Genitourinary Syndrome of Menopause (GSM)

The prevalence of urogenital symptoms in post menopause in the IMS study was 15%. It presents as vaginal dryness, pruritus vulvae, dyspareunia and urinary urgency. It is due to urogenital atrophy as a result of declining estrogen levels and may also present as recurrent urinary tract infections.

Local (vaginal) estrogen therapy offers significant relief with minimal systemic absorption. Vaginal DHEA and selective estrogen receptor modulators (SERMs) like ospemifene are the newer options.

Premature Ovarian Insufficiency

According to NFHS 2015-2016 data, 3.7% of the women are already in menopause by the age of 30–34 years; and the incidence rises to 8% for the age bracket of 35–39 years. Women with untreated premature menopause are at increased risk of developing osteoporosis, CVD, dementia, cognitive decline, Parkinson's and all-cause mortality and hence need MHT till the natural age of menopause

Other Potential Indications

- MHT may also be considered for osteoporosis prevention in women under 60 or within 10 years of menopause who are at high risk of developing Osteoporosis.
- It might also help improve quality of life by addressing symptoms like joint pain, mood swings, and sleep issues.
- It could potentially lower the risk of coronary heart disease and overall mortality, though it's not approved solely for this purpose. MHT is not to be used for the primary protection of CVD.

Right Timing

- Clearly define the timing of starting the MHT – Window of Opportunity: Less than 10 years of Menopause and less than 60 years of age.

Right Patient

- Determine the contraindications and evaluate the individual risk.

CONTRAINDICATIONS

- Undiagnosed vaginal bleeding
- Breast Cancer (Current, past or at high risk)
- CVD or Thromboembolic event (Current, recent or past or high risk)
- Hormone-dependent cancers (endometrial or ovarian)
- Active Liver disease
- Pregnancy

EVALUATION

Risk Assessment

- *Breast Cancer Risk Assessment tools:* These are the two most frequently used tools for Breast Cancer risk assessment. Those found to be at high risk, should not be offered MHT. Use the Gail score to assess the risk of developing breast cancer. It is available online and discussed elsewhere in this book.

- *CVD Risk Assessment:* Before initiating menopausal hormone therapy (MHT), a comprehensive cardiovascular disease (CVD) risk assessment is essential for all women.

Standard Risk Assessment Steps

- Comprehensive patient history
  - *Traditional factors:* Age, smoking status, blood pressure, cholesterol levels (total, HDL, LDL), diabetes status, physical activity level, diet, height, weight (BMI), and family history of premature CVD.
  - *Female-specific factors:* Age at menopause onset (early or premature menopause increases CVD risk), history of adverse pregnancy outcomes (e.g., preeclampsia, gestational diabetes), polycystic ovarian syndrome, and autoimmune conditions
- *Use of Formal Risk Calculators:* Use validated tools to estimate the 10-year CVD risk:
  - *ASCVD risk calculator (Pooled cohort equations)*: This tool is widely used to estimate the 10-year risk of atherosclerotic cardiovascular disease events (heart attack, stroke) for individuals aged 40 to 79. It is available online from the American College of Cardiology/American Heart Association (ACC/AHA).
  - *NAMS MenoPro App:* The Menopause Society (NAMS) offers a specific decision-support app that incorporates a woman's age, time since menopause, symptoms, and CVD risk factors to guide MHT decisions.
  - *WHO SEAR (WHO South-East Asia Region):* It is a colour coded chart. Available on WHO website.
  - *Laboratory-based charts:* These require information on age, sex, smoking status, systolic blood pressure, diabetes status, and total cholesterol values to estimate the 10-year CVD risk.
  - *Non-laboratory-based charts:* For areas where lab testing is limited, these charts can be used as a pre-screening tool. They rely on age, sex, smoking status, systolic blood pressure, and BMI (or waist circumference).

Risk	*ASVCD*	*WHO SEAR*	*MHT*
High	>10%	10–19%	Not recommended
Intermediate	5–10%	5–9%	Caution
Low	<5%	<5 %	Safe

Assessment – Clinical Examination

- Height and Weight – BMI
- Waist Circumference
- Blood Pressure and CVS
- Breast Examination
- *Pelvic Examination:*
  - Assess Physical Fitness
  - Assessment of Mood and Cognition
  - Ophthalmic Examination
  - Dental Check up
  - Assessment for Sarcopenia

Assessment – Investigations

- Complete Blood Picture
- LFT and KFT
- Lipid Profile
- Glycosylated Hemoglobin
- Thyroid Profile
- Vitamin D and B_{12}
- *Specific Investigations*
  - Whole Abdomen with TVS
  - Pap's Smear
  - Mammogram
  - Cardiac evaluation if needed
  - DEXA scan

Further targeted investigations can be conducted depending on the individualized risk assessment by history and examination.

FOLLOW-UP OF A WOMAN ON MHT

Follow-up Schedule

- *Initial Review (3 months):* The first check-up should occur about three months after starting MHT or changing the dose/formulation
- *Annual Reviews:* Even if the woman is accepting the MHT well, subsequent reviews should happen at least once a year.
- *As Needed:* The woman should be encouraged to come sooner if she experiences persistent symptoms, new or concerning side effects, or unscheduled vaginal bleeding.

At each review

- Assess Compliance
- Assess Symptoms and Efficacy
- Monitor for Side Effects
- Check Vitals and Lifestyle
- Review and Reassess Risk Profile
- Ensure Screening is Up-to-Date: Pap's Smear, Mammogram

Common side effects to be addressed at follow up visits:

- *Unscheduled or irregular bleeding with continuous combined EPT:* is a common occurrence, especially in the first 3–6 months of treatment (may occur in 60% of woman)

- Check for compliance and missed tablets
- Reassess the previous records - TVS and Pap's smear and medication history
- Reassure but if bleeding persists beyond 6 months or is heavy and continuous - she needs to be evaluated.

- *Breast Tenderness:* a very common side effect of MHT, particularly with regimens involving estrogen and progesterone.
  - Reassurance with advice to wait and see
  - Change of progesterone
  - Reducing the dose of estrogen
  - Switch regime
  - Change to transdermal route

SUGGESTED READING

1. Gail MH, Brinton LA, Byar DP, Corle DK, Green SB, Schairer C, et al. Projecting individualized probabilities of developing breast cancer for white females who are being examined annually. J Natl Cancer Inst. 1989;81(24):1879-86.
2. Goff Jr DC, Lloyd-Jones DM, Bennett G, Coady S, Conroy GM, Furberg CD, et al. 2013 ACC/AHA Guideline on the Assessment of Cardiovascular Risk: A Report of the American College of Cardiology/American Heart Association Task Force on Practice Guidelines. Circulation, 2013;129(25 Suppl 2):S49–S73.
3. International Institute for Population Sciences (IIPS) and ICF. 2017. National Family Health Survey (NFHS-4), 2015-16: India. Mumbai: IIPS.
4. International Menopause Society. (2016). 2016 IMS Recommendations on women's midlife health and menopause hormone therapy: an International Menopause Society Postion Statement.
5. Manson JE, Bassuk SS, Kaunitz AM, Pinkerton JV. The Women's Health Initiative trials of menopausal hormone therapy: lessons learned. Menopause. 2020;27(8):918-928.
6. Manson JE, Stuenkel CA, Barbieri RL, Pinkerton JV. Algorithm and mobile app for menopausal symptom management and hormonal/nonhormonal therapy decision making: a clinical decision-support tool from The North American Menopause Society. Menopause: The Journal of The North American Menopause Society, 2014;21(10):1039–45.
7. Meeta M, Digumarti L, Agarwal N, Vaze N, Shah R, Malik S. Clinical practice guidelines on menopause: An executive summary and recommendations: Indian menopause society 2019–2020. J Mid-lifeHealth 2020;11:55-95.
8. World Health Organization (2007). Prevention of cardiovascular disease: pocket guidelines for assessment and management of cardiovascular risk: (WHO/ISH cardiovascular risk prediction charts for the South-East Asia Region). World Health Organization.

3 CHAPTER

Prescribing MHT

Kiranjeet Kaur

PRESCRIBING MHT

Approach to a woman (40 years +) presenting with:

↓

Symptoms:
- Vasomotor- Hot flushes, night sweats
- Poor sleep
- Joint pains
- Central weight gain
- Irregular bleeding

Anxiety/Low mood
Cognitive Concerns
Low sex drive
Vaginal dryness

↓

Assess whether patient is pre/peri/postmenupausal

↓

Detailed history:
- Relevant gynae history- bleeding pattern, contraceptive use, past surgery e.g., hysterectomy/oophorectomy
- Co-morbidities- DVT/PE, breast/endometrial cancer, liver/thyroid disease, diabetes, HTN/ CVD, depression, osteoporosis
- Family history- CVD, osteoporosis/fractures, dementia, cancer
- Current medications; smoking

Midlife women general health assessment:
- CBC/Ferritin
- TSH
- FBG/HBAIC
- Lipid Profile
- RFT/LFT
- Vit-D in at risk woman
- Ultrasound Pelvis
- Pap-smear

Examination:
- Height and weight; Blood pressure
- Breast examination
- P/S and P/V

Patient care considerations

↓

Premenopause | Peri and early menopause | Postmenopause

General health/disease prevention and management:
- Lifestyle modification

↓

Contraceptive needs

↓

Management of:
- Menopausal symptoms
- Urogenital atrophy
- Prevention of osteoporosis

Hormone therapy (HT or MHT) remains the most effective treatment for moderate to severe menopausal symptoms and prevention of long-term estrogen deficiency effects in postmenopausal women.

ASSESS PATIENT CRITERIA BEFORE PRESCRIBING MHT

- Eligibility criteria/Indication
- Right window of opportunity
- Risk assessment/Rule out contraindications
- Right choice of MHT

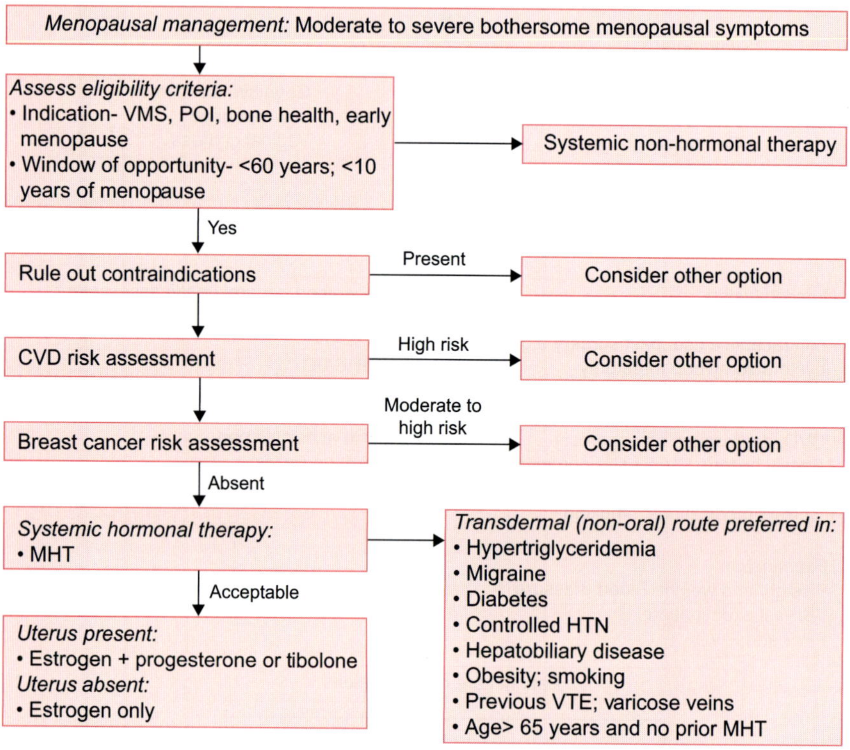

What to consider while making Right choice of MHT:

- Right Estrogen
- Right Progesterone
- Right Dose
- Right Route
- Right Regime
- Right Duration

RIGHT ESTROGEN

TABLE 1: Types of estrogens available.

17β-Estradiol Hemihydrate (E2)	*Estradiol Valerate (EV)*	*Conjugated Equine Estrogen (CEE)*	*Ethinyl Estradiol (EE)*
Biologically identical to endogenous human estradiol	Metabolized in liver to 17ß-estradiol and valeric acid	Mixture of estrone and equilin sulfate. (pregnant mares' urine)	Synthetic derivative of estradiol
Unconjugated, hence rapidly absorbed (micronized) through the lymphatic system and escapes first pass metabolism in liver	Extensive first pass metabolism in liver	Circulating estrone sulfate accumulates as a large precursor pool, is then continuously desulfated and converted to estradiol	Extensively conjugated, Resistant to metabolism
Minimal liver load	High liver load	2-3 times higher liver load	High first pass metabolism, cholestatic hepatotoxicity
Circulates in plasma as "free" estradiol		Prothrombotic effect-increased risk of VTE and Stroke	Increased risk of VTE and Stroke

RIGHT PROGESTERONE

Progesterone should be added to counteract endometrial proliferation due to unopposed estrogen if a woman has a uterus.

Most studies of the efficacy of progestins, including the Women's Health Initiative (WHI), have used *medroxy-progesterone acetate (MPA)*. Although MPA has proven efficacy for preventing endometrial hyperplasia, it appears to be associated with an excess risk of breast cancer, unfavorable effects on lipids and possibly coronary heart disease.

Natural oral micronized progesterone (NMP) is structurally identical to the progesterone secreted by the human ovary and is metabolically neutral (ie, does not negate the beneficial effects of estrogens on lipids). NMP and dydrogesterone do not appear to increase the risk of either breast cancer or cardiovascular disease.

LNG-IUS provide very high intrauterine but low systemic concentration of levonorgestrel; almost all women develop a non-proliferative, atrophic endometrium. LNG-IUS is an option if unable to tolerate oral progestins or in perimenopausal women who either need contraception, are having heavy bleeding, or both.

Tissue selective estrogen complexes (TSECs): Combination of a selective estrogen receptor modulator (SERM) and an estrogen. The SERM bazedoxifene prevents estrogen-induced endometrial hyperplasia so that administering a progestin is not necessary in women with a uterus (not available in India).

RIGHT DOSE

The most appropriate, lowest effective dose of systemic estrogen therapy should be used to provide benefit and minimize risks to achieve the therapeutic goal. The dosing regimen of progesterone depends on the potency of progesterone and the dose of estrogen used in the regimen.

TABLE 2: Dosage of different types of systemic estrogens used for MHT.

Estrogens	*Ultra-low dose*	*Low dose*	*Standard (Mid-range) dose*	*High Dose*
CEE (oral)-mg	0.15	0.3, 0.45	0.625	1.25
17ß-estradiol (oral)-mg	–	0.5	1.0	1.5-2.0
Estradiol Valerate (oral)-mg	–	0.5	1.0	2.0
Estriol-mg	1.0-2.0			
Estradiol gel- mg		0.5	1.0	1.5
Estradiol hemihydrate (transdermal gel)-mg	0.375	0.75 (1 pump)	1.5 (2 pumps)	2.25-3.0 (3-4 pumps)
17ß-estradiol (transdermal patch)-mcg/day	14	25 mcg/day	50 mcg/day	75-100 mcg/day
Estradiol transdermal spray (mg/spray)	-	1.53 (1 spray)	3.06 (2 sprays)	4.50 (3 sprays)

Low-dose estrogen is effective for hot flashes in many women and is associated with fewer side effects. CEE 0.625 mg is considered standard-dose estrogen as it has been used by most studies on safety and efficacy. Similarly effective doses of other estrogens for the treatment of VMS as 0.625 mg of CEE include 1mg micronized 17ß-estradiol, 0.75 mg 17ß-estradiol transdermal gel, 0.5 mg 17ß-estradiol transdermal patch and 5 mcg of EE. The lowest-dose patch containing 0.014 mg of 17ß-estradiol is approved for the prevention of osteoporosis.

The usual dose of NMP is 200 mg/day for 12-14 days/month (vaginally 100 mg/day) is adequate for prevention of endometrial hyperplasia when combined with continuous estrogen in sequential HT. While usual dose of NMP in continuous HT is 100 mg/day, a regimen of 200 mg/day continuously is sometimes used to prevent bleeding and avoid endometrial proliferation. Women taking lower doses of estrogen (e.g., 0.014 mg transdermal estradiol) require very little progestin (a 12-day course every 6 to 12 months).

TABLE 3

Progesterone	*With low dose E*	*With mid or highest dose E*
Cyclical progesterone (sequential): 12-14 days /month for endometrial protection.		
Natural Micronized Progesterone (oral)	200 mg	200 mg
Dydroprogesterone (oral)	5 mg	10 mg
Norethisterone acetate (oral)	1.5–2.5 mg	2.5–5 mg
Medroxyprogesterone acetate (oral)	5 mg	5–10 mg
Continuous progesterone: daily dose for endometrial protection		
Natural Micronized Progesterone (oral)	100 mg	100 mg (may not be adequate with high dose E)
Dydrogesterone (oral)	5 mg	10 mg
Norethisterone acetate (oral)	0.1 mg with 0.5 mg estradiol 0.5 mg with 1.0 mg estradiol	1.0–2.5 mg
Medroxyprogesterone acetate (oral)	2.5 mg	2.5-5 mg
LNG-IUS	Releases 20 mcg/ day	

RIGHT ROUTE

- *Systemic estrogen* can be prescribed as oral drugs, transdermal gels, sprays and patches, or as vaginal rings with systemic absorption is used for widespread symptoms (VMS, sleep disturbance, mood, and bone effect).
- *Local (vaginal) therapy* (low-dose vaginal estrogen creams, tablets, rings) primarily for GSM (vaginal dryness, dyspareunia, urinary symptoms). Because systemic absorption is minimal, risks are lower.
- *Transdermal estrogen* (patch/gels) may have a more favorable risk profile compared with oral, particularly regarding VTE and stroke risk (bypassing first-pass hepatic metabolism).

RIGHT REGIME

HT Options for Systemic Therapy

- Estrogen
- Progesterone
- Combination of Estrogen and Progesterone
- SERMs- Bazedoxifene + CEE; Ospemifene (not available in India)
- Tibolone (STEAR- selective tissue estrogen activity regulator)

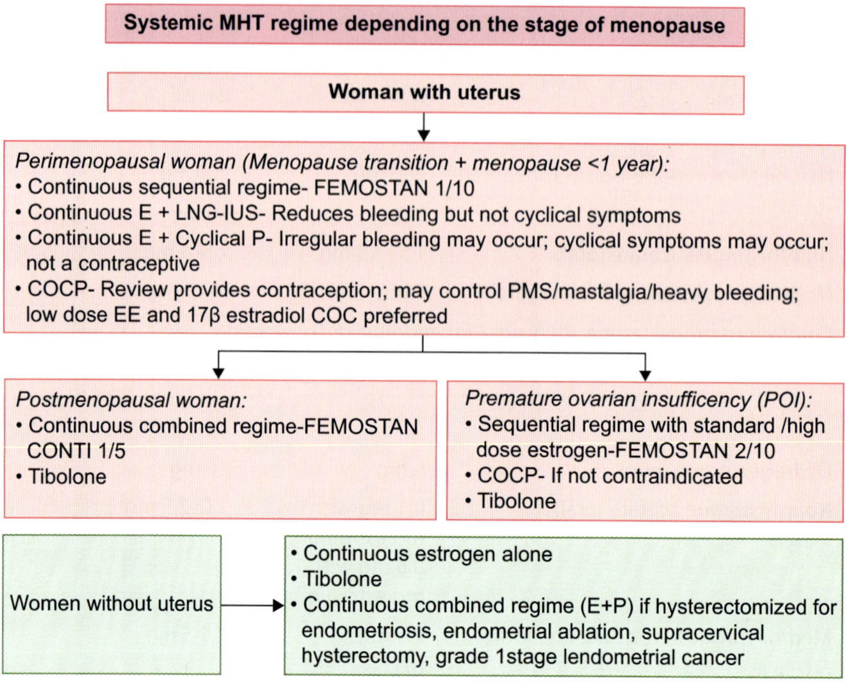

MHT FORMULATIONS AVAILABLE IN INDIA

Estrogen

- *Oral route:* CEE 0.3/0.625 mg; 17ß-estradiol 1 mg/2 mg; Estradiol valerate 1 mg/2 mg
- *Transdermal route:* 17ß-estradiol 1.5 mg per 2.5 gm gel; Estradiol spray 1.53 mg/actuation (8.1 mL/56 sprays)

Progesterone

- Dydrogesterone- oral 10 mg
- Natural Micronized Progesterone- oral/vaginal 100/200/300/400 mg
- Levonorgestrel Intrauterine Device- 52 mg releases 20 mcg/day (LNG-IUS)

Combination of Estrogen and Progesterone

Continuous Sequential formulation—(tablets have to be taken every single day).

- 17ß-estradiol 1 mg + dydrogesterone 10 mg (perimenopause) when a woman expects regular periods
- 17ß-estradiol 2 mg + dydrogesterone 10 mg (POI)

Continuous Combined formulation (Tablets have to be taken every single day.)

- 17β-estradiol 1mg + dydrogesterone 5mg (postmenopause) when the patient does not want periods after menopause.

Tibolone: 2.5 mg/day

Fixed Dose Formulations	
Continuous Sequential	• 17β-estradiol 1 mg + dydrogesterone 10 mg - FEMOSTAN 1/10 All 28 tablets have estradiol valerate, and last 14 tablets have estradiol valerate and dydrogesterone together. Patient has to take 1 tablet every single day, no pill-free interval • 17ß-estradiol 2mg + dydrogesterone 10 mg - FEMOSTAN 2/10
Continuous Combined	17β-estradiol 1 mg + dydrogesterone 5mg Femostan Conti 1/5 All 28 tablets have 17 b estradiol 1 mg and dydrogesterone 5 mg together. Patient has to take 1 tablet every single day, no pill-free interval
LIVIAL	2.5 mg/day- Tibolone
DUAVE	0.45 mg CEE + 20 mg Bazedoxifene (not available in India)

RIGHT DURATION

- The decision regarding duration of treatment and when to stop hormone therapy must be considered in the context of the individualized risk-benefit profile, as well as the woman's personal preference.
- According to available data of WHI, the longest adequately powered, blinded RCT, is limited to 5 to 7 years of therapy.
- In women with POI, hormone therapy is recommended at least until the average age of menopause (50–52 years of age).
- Hormone therapy does not need to be routinely discontinued in women aged older than 60 or 65 years.
- Long-term use of hormone therapy may be considered in a healthy woman at low risk of CVD and breast cancer with persistent VMS, including woman older than 60 years, though limited by insufficient evidence on safety, risks and benefit. Continuation of hormone therapy beyond 60 years is reasonable after appropriate counselling, risk stratification, clear benefit and shared decision making.
- Long-term use of hormone therapy may be considered for woman at increased risk of fracture for whom other fracture-prevention therapies are not appropriate.

Potential Risks and Benefits of MHT

- Overall, increased absolute risks associated with estrogen-progesterone therapy and estrogen-only therapy is rare (<10/10,000/y), including risk for VTE and gall bladder disease.

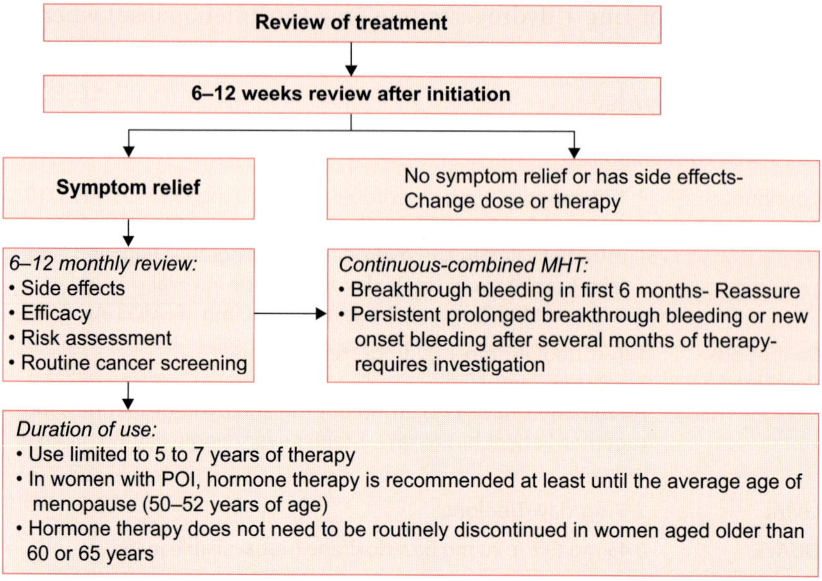

- There is a rare increased risk for stroke and breast cancer with estrogen-progesterone therapy.
- There is an increased risk of endometrial hyperplasia and endometrial cancer if estrogen is used unopposed.
- There is a reduced absolute risk for all-cause mortality, fracture, diabetes mellitus (EPT and ET) and breast cancer (ET) in women aged younger than 60 years.
- Common adverse effects of hormone therapy include nausea, bloating, weight gain, fluid retention, mood swings (progesterone-related), breakthrough bleeding, headaches and breast tenderness.

KEY POINTS

- Start when symptoms are bothersome to the woman, not merely because of menopause per se.
- The sooner after menopause you initiate HT (within ~10 yrs, age<60 years) in a suitable woman, the more favorable the benefit-risk balance.
- Use lowest effective dose, tailor to the route and formulation (transdermal preferred in some higher-risk situations).
- Include progestogen in women with a uterus for endometrial protection when using systemic estrogen.
- Always engage in shared decision-making- inform the woman of benefits, risks, alternatives, and her preferences matter.
- Monitoring is essential- regular review, reassessment of risks/benefits and symptoms.
- For women beyond age 65 or >10 yrs post-menopause, evidence of benefit is less strong and risks higher; do not assume indefinite therapy without review.
- Lifestyle measures (smoking cessation, physical activity, healthy diet) remain foundational- HT does not replace these.

SUGGESTED READING

1. Baker VL. Alternatives to oral estrogen replacement. Transdermal patches, percutaneous gels, vaginal creams and rings, implants, other methods of delivery. Obstet Gynecol Clin North Am. 1994;21(2):271-97.
2. Eden J. The endometrial and breast safety of menopausal hormone therapy containing micronised progesterone: a short review. Aust N Z J ObstetGynaecol 2017;57:12-15.
3. Ettinger B, Ensrud KE, Wallace R, Johnson KC, Cummings SR, Yankov V, Vittinghoff E, Grady D. Effects of ultralow-dose transdermal estradiol on bone mineral density: a randomized clinical trial. Obstet Gynecol. 2004;104(3): 443-51.
4. Johnson SR, Ettinger B, Macer JL, Ensrud KE, Quan J, Grady D. Uterine and vaginal effects of unopposed ultralow-dose transdermal estradiol. Obstet Gynecol. 2005;105(4):779-87.
5. Kim JE, Chang JH, Jeong MJ, et al. A systematic review and meta-analysis of effects of menopausal hormone therapy on cardiovascular diseases.Sci Rep 2020;10:20631.
6. Manson JE, Bassuk SS, Kaunitz AM, Pinkerton JV. The Women's Health Initiative trials of menopausal hormone therapy: lessons learned. Menopause. 2020;27(8):918-928.
7. Manson JE, Chlebowski RT, Stefanick ML, et al. Menopausal hormone therapy and health outcomes during the intervention and extended poststopping phases of the Women's Health Initiative randomized trials. JAMA 2013;310:1353-1368.
8. Manson JE, Flores VA, Pal L. (2021). Hormone Therapy in Menopause: Concepts, Controversies, and Approach to Treatment. Endocrine Reviews, 42(6), 720–752. https://doi.org/10.1210/endrev/bnab011
9. Meeta, Digumarti L, Agarwal N, Vaze N, Shah R, Malik S, Clinical Practice Guidelines on Menopause: Indian menopause society 2020.
10. Meeta M, Digumarti L, Agarwal N, Vaze N, Shah R,Malik S. Clinical practice guidelines on menopause: An executive summary and recommendations: Indian menopause society 2019–2020. J Mid-lifeHealth 2020;11:55-95.
11. Menopause: The Journal of The North American Menopause Society, Vol. 29, No. 7, pp. 767-794.
12. RJ Baber, N Panay, A Fenton the IMS Writing Group 2016 IMS. Recommendations on women's midlife health and menopause hormone therapy, Climacteric, 2016;19:2:109-150.
13. Stevenson JC, Cust MP, Gangar KF, Hillard TC, Lees B, Whitehead MI. Effects of transdermal versus oral hormone replacement therapy on bone density in spine and proximal femur in postmenopausal women. Lancet. 1990; 336(8710):265-9.
14. Stute P, Neulen J, Wildt L. The impact of micronized progesterone on the endometrium: a systematic review. Climacteric 2016;19:316-328.

4 CHAPTER

HRT in Breast Cancer Survivor

Anita Kant, Amrita Razdan Kaul

HRT IN BREAST CANCER SURVIVOR

Menopausal symptoms are common and more severe in breast cancer survivors because of treatment-induced ovarian failure. MHT (also known as HRT) in breast cancer survivors is a nuanced and evolving area. Breast cancer is a contraindication for the use of Systemic Replacement Therapy (HRT) due to the increased risk of recurrence in both the ipsi and contralateral breast carcinoma. This statement is based on the HABITS study opened in 1996 (Hormonal replacement therapy after breast cancer - is it safe?) trial. Tibolone was associated with an increased risk of recurrence (HR = 1.64, 95% CI 0.99-2.72). Lupo et al. (2015) proposed a stepwise algorithm for the treatment of vasomotor symptoms, starting with non-hormonal therapy. If there is insufficient improvement, a comprehensive discussion should follow regarding the current evidence for and against HRT with shared decision-making with the patient for Control of Menopausal Symptoms, like vasomotor symptoms, arthralgia, sleeping disorders, genitourinary symptoms, osteopenia/osteoporosis, prevention of cardiovascular disease, risk of recurrence of breast cancer, and quality of life desired by the patient.

NONHORMONAL THERAPIES

They are advised as first-line therapy for vasomotor and other menopausal symptoms in those who have completed their treatment for breast cancer.

SSRIs/SNRIs Selective Serotonin Reuptake Inhibitors (SSRIs) are a class of antidepressants, but can be used for the treatment of hot flashes. They have also been shown to be safe in women with (a history of) breast cancer. Venlafaxine, Paroxetine, and Citalopram show modest efficacy while treating vasomotor symptoms. Paroxetine should be avoided with Tamoxifen due to CYP2D6 inhibition, as this enzyme metabolizes Tamoxifen to its active form.

Gabapentin and Pregabalin: Gabapentin was developed for the treatment of epileptic seizures but is also used for neuropathic pain and off-label for chronic low back pain or radicular pain. Effective for hot flashes, particularly nocturnal symptoms. Gabapentin has similar effects to venlafaxine.

Clonidine has central α-adrenergic activity and may be used in the treatment of hypertension. Clonidine reduces vasomotor symptoms. Side effects may include drowsiness and dry mouth.

Oxybutynin: Oxybutynin is commonly used to treat overactive bladder and urinary incontinence. Placebo-controlled trials have shown that 73% of patients had fewer vasomotor symptoms after 12 weeks of treatment with oxybutynin 15 mg once daily

Neurokinin receptor antagonists: Elinzanetant and Fezolinetant are non-hormonal dual neurokinin-1,3 receptor antagonists. Placebo-controlled trials have already shown safety and effectiveness in reducing vasomotor symptoms in menopausal women without a history of breast cancer. A randomized phase III study is currently underway to evaluate the effect in women with (a history of) breast cancer.

Cognitive-behavioral therapy and Tai Chi: Arico et al. (2016) suggest that cognitive-behavioral therapy is an effective treatment for insomnia in breast cancer patients, with improvements in mood, overall and physical fatigue, and quality of life.

Lifestyle modifications: Regular exercise, weight management, and giving up smoking may help. These are all universally recommended, as they lead to overall health improvement.

Acupuncture and hypnotherapy: A meta-analysis suggests that acupuncture is a safe non-pharmacological option capable to significantly reduce arthralgia.

Osteopenia and osteoporosis: Lifestyle interventions, calcium, and vitamin D intake Adjuvant treatment (in the form of chemotherapy, GnRH agonists, or AIs) can lead to bone loss, potentially resulting in osteoporosis and fractures. The prevention and treatment of osteoporosis in women with a history of breast carcinoma are similar to those in women without breast cancer. Bisphosphonates are safe for long- term use and are effective in reducing the risk of bone-related events, such as pathological fractures and spinal cord compression. This is particularly important because the incidence of bone-related events is highest in breast cancer patients compared with all other cancer patients.

Topic vaginal non-hormonal treatment: Due to adjuvant endocrine treatment, chemotherapy and/or premature ovarian failure, women with a history of breast cancer often experience more severe and prolonged symptoms of the genitourinary syndrome of menopause than those with natural menopause Symptoms of the genitourinary syndrome may include vaginal dryness, irritation, itching, recurrent infections, urinary urgency, and dyspareunia. Treatment should be individualized and there is no one-size-fits-all approach. Non-hormonal options for menopausal genitourinary syndrome include daily use of vaginal moisturizing creams, lubricants during sexual activity, topical application of xylocaine gel, pelvic floor therapy and dilators/vibrators. Dynamic quadripolar radiofrequency (DQRF) is a novel technique rapidly gaining attention for improvements in vulvovaginal aesthetics, sexual satisfaction and relief of symptoms caused by vulvovaginal atrophy. However, the technique has not been studied in women with a history of breast cancer.

Key Points from Recent Evidence and Guidelines

Nonhormonal therapies (e.g., SSRIs/SNRIs, gabapentin, clonidine, cognitive behavioral therapy, lifestyle modifications) are first-line for vasomotor and other menopausal symptoms in breast cancer survivors.

TABLE 1: Nonhormonal options for menopausal symptoms in breast cancer survivors.

Therapy/ Intervention	Symptoms Targeted	Efficacy/Notes	Key Considerations
SSRIs/SNRIs	Vasomotor (Hot flashes)	Modest reduction infrequency/ severity; Venlafaxine, Citalopram, Escitalopram	Paroxetine/ fluoxetine inhibit CYP2D6—avoid with Tamoxifen
Gabapentin/ Pregablin	Vasomotor, sleep	Effective specially for nocturnal symptoms	Sedation, dizziness may limit use
Clonidine	Vasomotor	Mild benefit, less effective than above	Hypotension, dry mouth, constipation
Oxybutynin	Vasomotor	Some evidence for hot flash reduction	Anticholinergic side effects
Desvenlafaxine	Vasomotor	RCTs show efficacy for hot flashes	Similar side effect profile to other SNRIs
Cognitive Behavioral Therapy (CBT)	Vasomotor, mood, sleep	Reduces symptom bother and improves coping	No pharmacologic side effects
Lifestyle(Exercise, weight loss, smoking cessation)	Vasomotor, general	Modest benefit, overall health improvement	Safe, universally recommended

PATIENT GROUP RECOMMENDATION FOR MHT

- HR-positive breast cancer Generally avoid; consider only in exceptional cases after multidisciplinary review.
- HR-negative breast cancer May be considered if symptoms are severe and nonhormonal options have failed, after risk-benefit discussion.
- Local (vaginal) estrogen May be considered for severe genitourinary symptoms, especially with tamoxifen, caution with aromatase inhibitors.

TOPICAL HORMONAL TREATMENT

Topical estrogens may be considered for women with a history of breast cancer for genitourinary symptoms not responding to non- hormonal preparations. There are no large randomized controlled trials demonstrating the safety of topical estrogen therapy in breast cancer patients. However, several observational studies have shown no significant difference in recurrence. The use of ultralow-dose 0.005% estriol vaginal gel does not significantly influence oestrogens, FSH, and LH levels in women with breast cancer receiving Aromatase Inhibitors. A randomized trial suggests a significant improvement in signs of vulvovaginal atrophy with the use of ultra-low dose 0.005% estriol vaginal gel compared with placebo. There are no studies on long-term results or the risk of recurrence.

Vaginal dehydroepiandrosterone (DHEA), estriol and oral ospemifene are alternatives to local estrogen therapy when non-hormonal measures do not provide adequate relief. DHEA is a precursor of androgens and did not cause a significant increase in blood levels of estrogen and androgens in studies of postmenopausal women. More studies are needed to establish safety, particularly in patients with breast cancer or a history of breast cancer.

TABLE 2: Local estrogen options for GSM in breast cancer survivors.

Product/ Preparation	*Typical dose/ regimen*	*Systemic absorption*	*Evidence on recurrence risk*	*Key recommendations*
Vaginal estradiol tablet (10mcg)	1 tab daily for 2 weeks, then 2 times a week	Minimal	No increased recurrence specially with tamoxifen	Preferred for minimal systemic exposure; Cautionwith aromatase inhibitors
Vaginal Estradiol cream	0.5 mg daily for 2-3 weeks, then 2-3 times per week	Minimal	No significant increase in recurrence risk	Often used in Europe, not available everywhere
Vaginal Estradiol ring	7.5 mcg/24 h, replaced after 90 days	Minimal	No significant increase in recurrence risk	Convenient for long term use
Vaginal conjugated estrogen cream	0.5 mg daily for 2 weeks, then 2–3 times a wk	Slightly higher but still low	Use lowest effective dose for shortest duration	Use lowest effective dose, shortest duration
Prasterone (DHEA) vaginal insert	6.5 mg daily	Minimal	Limited data in breast cancer survivors	Not first line, consider only after specialist input

Ospemifene is a SERM developed for the treatment of genitourinary symptoms and is not thought to have any estrogenic effects on the breast. However, it is not yet approved for use in breast cancer patients because there are no studies to prove its safety. Its use is not recommended by international guidelines.

Key Points from Recent Evidence and Guidelines

Local estrogen for women with severe GSM unresponsive to nonhormonal options can be considered. Alternatives to local estrogen include nonhormonal moisturizers/lubricants.

Recent findings: There is a discordance between randomized and observational data regarding the risk of systemic menopausal hormone therapy and breast cancer recurrence; hormone receptor status is significant to recurrence risk in this setting. The systemic absorption of local oestrogen is not a consistent surrogate marker for cancer recurrence, and clinical data have not demonstrated a consistent increase in the risk of cancer recurrence with local therapy.

SUMMARY

- Systemic MHT (oral or transdermal estrogen, with or without progestogen) is generally contraindicated in women with hormone receptor-positive breast cancer. Meta analysis and RCTs show an increased risk of recurrence (HR 1.5–1.8).
- Nonhormonal therapies are first-line for both vasomotor and genito-urinary symptoms.
- Choice of agent should be individualized based on symptom profile, comorbidities, and drug interactions (notably, avoid strong CYP2D6 inhibitors with tamoxifen).
- For GSM, start with nonhormonal moisturizers/lubricants; consider local estrogen only if symptoms are severe and refractory, after multidisciplinary discussion.

SUGGESTED READING

1. Arico D, Raggi A, Ferri R. Cognitive Behavioral Therapy For Insomnia In Breast Cancer Survivors: A Review Of The Literature. Front Psychol. 2016;7:1162.
2. Barton DL, Shuster LT, Dockter T, et al. Systemic and local effects of vaginal dehydroepiandrosterone (DHEA): NCCTG N10C1 (Alliance). Support Care Cancer. 2018;26:1335–1343.
3. Cagnacci A, Xholli A, Venier M. Ospemifene in the management of vulvar and vaginal atrophy: focus on the assessment of patient acceptability and ease of use. patient prefer adherence. 2020;14:55–62.

4. Chen L, Lin CC, Huang TW, et al. Effect of acupuncture on aromatase inhibitor-induced arthralgia in patients with breast cancer: a meta-analysis of randomized controlled trials. Breast. 2017;33:132–138.
5. Chubak J, Bowles EJA, Yu O, et al. Breast cancer recurrence in relation to antidepressant use. Cancer Causes Control. 2016;27:125–136. doi: 10.1007/s10552-015-0689-y.
6. Coleman R, Hadji P, Body JJ, et al. Bone health in cancer: ESMO Clinical Practice Guidelines. Ann Oncol. 2020;31:1650–1663.
7. Elbiss HM, Rafaqat W, Khan KS. The effect of dynamic quadripolar radiofrequency on genitourinary atrophy and sexual satisfaction: A systematic review and meta-analysis. Medicine (Baltimore) 2022;101:e30960.
8. Friedman GD, Udaltsova N, Habel LA. Norepinephrine antagonists and cancer risk. Int J Cancer. 2011;128:737–738.
9. Go J, Park S, Kim KS, et al. Risk of osteoporosis and fracture in long-term breast cancer survivors. Korean J Clin Oncol. 2020;16:39–45.
10. Hirschberg AL, Sanchez-Rovira P, Presa-Lorite J, et al. Efficacy and safety of ultra-low dose 0.005% estriol vaginal gel for the treatment of vulvovaginal atrophy in postmenopausal women with early breast cancer treated with nonsteroidal aromatase inhibitors: a phase ii, randomized, double-blind, placebo- controlled trial. Menopause. 2020;27:526–534.
11. Holmberg L, Anderson H. HABITS (hormonal replacement therapy after breast cancer—is it safe?), a randomised comparison: trial stopped. Lancet. 2004;363:453–455.
12. Lupo M, Dains JE, Madsen LT. J Adv Pract Oncol. Hormone Replacement Therapy: An Increased Risk of Recurrence and Mortality for Breast Cancer Patients. 2015;6:322–330.
13. Perez-Lopez FR, Phillips N, Vieira-Baptista P, et al. Management of postmenopausal vulvovaginal atrophy: recommendations of the International Society for the Study of Vulvovaginal Disease. Gynecol Endocrinol. 2021; 37:746–752.
14. Sanchez-Rovira P, Hirschberg AL, Gil-Gil M, et al. A Phase II Prospective, Randomized, Double-Blind, Placebo-Controlled and Multicenter Clinical Trial to Assess the Safety of 0.005% Estriol Vaginal Gel in Hormone Receptor-Positive Postmenopausal Women with Early Stage Breast Cancer in Treatment with Aromatase Inhibitor in the Adjuvant Setting. Oncologist. 2020;25:e1846–e1854.
15. Shan D, Zou L, Liu X, et al. Efficacy and safety of gabapentin and pregabalin in patients with vasomotor symptoms: a systematic review and meta-analysis. Am J Obstet Gynecol. 2020;222:564–579.e12.
16. Simon JA, Anderson RA, Ballantyne E, et al. Efficacy and safety of elinzanetant, a selective neurokinin-1,3 receptor antagonist for vasomotor symptoms: a dose-finding clinical trial (SWITCH-1). Menopause. 2023;30:239–246.
17. Simon JA, Gaines T, LaGuardia KD. Extended-release oxybutynin therapy for vasomotor symptoms in women: a randomized clinical trial. Menopause. 2016;23:1214–1221.
18. Sismondi P, Kimmig R, Kubista E, et al. Effects of tibolone on climacteric symptoms and quality of life in breast cancer patients—data from liberate trial. Maturitas. 2011;70:365–372.

19. Trower M, Anderson RA, Ballantyne E, et al. Effects of Nt-814, a dual neurokinin 1 and 3 receptor antagonist, on vasomotor symptoms in postmenopausal women: a placebo-controlled, randomized trial. Menopause. 2020;27:498–505.
20. Villa P, Tagliaferri V, Amar ID, et al. Local ultra-low-dose estriol gel treatment of vulvo-vaginal atrophy: efficacy and safety of long-term treatment. Gynecol Endocrinol. 2020;36:535–539. doi: 10.1080/09513590.2019.1702016.

5 CHAPTER

MHT in Patients with Hypertension or Diabetes

Bipasa Sen

Hormone therapy has always been a topic of controversy, confusion, myth-producing, as well as the center of overdependence or criticism, especially since the landmark WHI study in 2002.

The reanalysis of WHI data and many further studies and trials have pointed to a single direction - "individualization of Hormone Therapy" to get the women to benefit and no negative impact from it. Hormone therapy has to be individualized according to age, race, ethnicity, sociodemography and cultural factors and also according to the symptoms, needs, priority and co-morbidities of each beneficiary. Hormone therapy and its relation to co-morbidities like hypertension and diabetes should always be discussed as per risk risk-benefit assessment of each individual.

THE 5Ws OF PRESCRIBING MENOPAUSAL HORMONE THERAPY

(MHT – Previously called Hormone Replacement Therapy or HRT – which is now applicable in case of premature ovarian insufficiency or POI)

The White Paper published by the International Menopause Society at the Melbourne IMS Conference in October 2024 stressed on 5Ws for prescribing MHT, which include:

1. Who is MHT for
2. What types & doses of MHT
3. When should MHT be started and stopped
4. Why is MHT important
5. Where can MHT be accessed

Out of these 5Ws, the first one points towards absolute indication of Hormone Therapy, which are bothersome vasomotor symptoms and genitourinary syndrome. In the USA and Australia, Osteoporosis prevention also falls under the primary indication.

Many other women might benefit from Hormone Therapy, for whom it is not indicated according to the label. Under this category come many co-morbidities, including hypertension and diabetes. The second point in 5Ws - i.e. what types of MHT indicate estrogen and progesterone in different regimes and routes. Tibolone or SERM may be another option.

The Beneficial Effects of Estrogen to protect Women from Cardiovascular Emergencies include :

- Estrogen increases endothelial nitric oxide synthetase level – thus increasing potent vasodilator Nitric Oxide (NO) – resulting in vasodilatation. Nitric Oxide is involved in the regulation of blood pressure, platelet function, inhibition of vascular smooth muscle proliferation and expression of adhesion molecules.
- Estrogen reduces the release of Endothelin – 1, which is a family of peptides synthesized by Endothelial cells and acts in a paracrine fashion on smooth muscle cells to cause vasoconstriction.
- Post menopausal oral estrogen replacement results in lowering of PAI – 1 and E-Selectin in hypercholesterolaemic women.
- Decrease in cell adhesion molecules E- E-Selectin and VCAM – 1 have also been observed in healthy post menopausal women with both oral and transdermal HRT- suggestive of a reduction in vascular inflammatory changes.
- Estradiol inhibits Calcium influx in vascular smooth muscle and reduces intracellular free calcium in isolated cardiac myocytes. Thus, estrogen promotes vasodilatation, which benefits arterial function.
- A reduction in the activity of angiotensin-converting enzyme has been reported with both oral and transdermal HRT. Thus estrogen impacts on Renin-Angiotensin-Aldosterone System (RAAS), causing a beneficial effect in terms of CVD risk. The progesterone drosperinone, with its antimineralocorticoid effects, also influences RAAS. HRT containing transdermal estrogen and drospirenone results in a significant reduction in blood pressure in women with mild hypertension. Natural micronized progesterone generally does not raise BP. Synthetic progesterone, like Medroxyprogesterone acetate, might blunt estrogen's beneficial vascular effects.
- Estrogen improves lipid profile, homocysteine, fibrinogen; protects against the toxic effects of Oxidised LDL and thus helps in cardiovascular disease prevention.

MHT AND HYPERTENSION

- Hormone therapy with standard agents like estradiol valerate or conjugated equine estrogen has effect on blood pressure and can be given if the patient has controlled hypertension.
- However, ethinyl estradiol used in oral contraceptive pill has 4 times higher potency of estrogen and may cause deep vein thrombosis.
- In 11 of 13 studies with Transdermal Estrogen, blood pressure was reduced with MHT.
- Menopausal HT can improve in recently developed hypertension, often leading to an enhanced response to antihypertensive drugs.

- In case of aggressive postmenopausal hypertension, the option to initiate transdermal hormone therapy should be discussed with a cardiologist.
- Oral HRT may cause mild BP elevation in women with preexisting hypertension, but transdermal estradiol has a neutral or even beneficial effect on BP and Endothelial function.
- However, MHT is not indicated for the primary prevention of Cardiac disease.
- MHT is contraindicated in established coronary artery disease and uncontrolled hypertension.

EVIDENCE SUMMARY

- Large studies (WHI, HERS) found no major increase in hypetension risk with HRT overall, but route and formulation matter. Transdermal route preferred. Of the progesterone part of HRT, micronized progesterone and dydrogesterone preferred.
- KEEPS Trial showed that oral 0.45 mg conjugated equine estrogen or transdermal estradiol patch, along with cyclical micronized progesterone 200mg per day for 12 days, if given within 36 months of menopause, does not raise blood pressure.
- ELITE Trial showed that HRT containing 1mg of estradiol causes less progression of carotid intima media thickness if given within 6 yrs of menopause or in less than 60 yrs age group.

MONITORING AND SAFETY CHECKLIST FOR HRT

- Avoid oral estrogen in women with preexisting moderate hypertension.
- Avoid synthetic progesterone like medroxyprogesterone acetate.
- Transdermal estradiol patch plus oral micronized progesterone/ dydrogesterone preferred.
- Vaginal estrogen is always safe.
- Before starting HRT, check BP, assess CVD risk, BMI, Lipid profile and Glucose.
- Recheck BP after 6–12 weeks and adjust estrogen dose if required.
- Annually review symptoms, BP, breast and endometrial health.
- If persistent hypertension (≥160/100 mm Hg despite control) – stop HRT.

Algorithm: HRT in Hypertensive Women

- *Assess the woman:* Review the indication for HRT (vasomotor symptoms/ urogenital atrophy)
- Evaluate Blood Pressure and CVD Risk
  - If controlled BP (140/90 mm Hg) – proceed
  - If mild to moderate hypertension (140-159/90-99 mm Hg) – initiate HRT and optimize BP control.

- Uncontrolled hypertension (≥160/100 mm Hg) – defer HRT until BP is controlled (stroke risk).

- Choose the safest route :
  - Transdermal estrogen (patch/gel/spray) preferred.
  - Avoid oral estrogen as it increases hepatic angiotensinogen.
  - Vaginal estrogen – safe at all BP levels.
- Select an appropriate regimen
  - If uterus absent (except in hysterectomy due to endometriosis) – estrogen-only HRT.
  - If uterus present – combined regimen of estrogen and micronized progesterone.
- Initiate and monitor :
  - Baseline – record BP, BMI, Lipid Profile, Glucose.
  - After 6 – 12 weeks – recheck BP, assess symptoms.
  - Every 6 – 12 months – monitor BP, review HRT need, breast exam, and endometrial health.
- Continue/adjust/stop
  - BP Stable and symptom improved – continue HRT in lowest effective dose.
  - Mild BP increased – adjust antihypertensive / lower estrogen dose./
  - Persistent uncontrolled BP – discontinue HRT.
- Adjunct measures
  - Maintain a healthy weight, diet, and exercise.
  - Limit salt and alcohol intake.
  - Control Lipids and Glucose.
  - Consider non-hormonal options (SSRI, Gabapentine, Clonidine) if HRT is contraindicated.

Effect of HRT on Diabetes

- Glucose Metabolism :
  - Estrogen improves carbohydrate, insulin metabolism, reducing fasting glucose and insulin levels, improves insulin clearance and insulin sensitivity.
  - Estrogen enhances insulin secretion, glucose disposal, and increases the effectiveness of glucose and may also reduce the risk of type 2 Diabetes Mellitus by 30%.
- Lipid Profile
  - Estrogen raises HDL and lowers LDL and total cholesterol and thus controls dyslipidaemia.
  - Oral estrogen can raise triglycerides; transdermal estrogen has less effect.
  - For the progesterone part – dydrogesterone and natural micronized progesterone have a neutral effect on lipid profile.

- Body fat distribution and waist circumference:
  - Estrogen (through estrogen receptor alpha) prevents postmenopausal increase in central (android) fat and helps maintain gynecoid fat distribution – thus improves insulin resistance and reduces waist circumference and also inhibits the interactions among abdominal adiposity, hormones, insulin resistance, hyperinsulinemia, blood pressure and atherogenic lipid profile.
  - Thus, better control of type 2 Diabetes Mellitus is possible while on HRT.
  - There is a lack of evidence on the use of MHT in type 1 Diabetes.

PREFERRED REGIMENS

- Transdermal estrogen preferred for glucose metabolism, lipids and thrombotic risk.
- In the presence of an intact uterus, add micronized progesterone or dydrogesterone for their neutral effect on lipid profile.

MONITORING

- Regular checkup of BP, Glucose, Lipids and HBA1C needed.
- Estrogen/Progesterone levels are not traditionally measured. The improvement in the Menopause Rating Scale indicates adequate response.

KEY TAKEAWAYS

- HRT can be safely used in post menopausal women with controlled hypertension or type 2 Diabetes Mellitus, considering appropriate dose, regimen, duration, route and time of initiation.
- Regular monitoring is needed.
- Estrogen in HRT modestly improves glucose metabolism, insulin metabolism and lipid profile – especially with transdermal estrogen along with natural micronized progesterone or dydrogesterone due to their lipid neutral status.
- Individualization with shared decision-making is recommended.
- Cardiovascular and thrombotic risk must always be assessed before initiation and during therapy.

SUGGESTED READING

1. American Diabetes Association (ADA) 2025 Standards of Care.
2. European Menopause and Andropause Society (EMAS) 2022 Position Statement.
3. Hugh S Taylor, Lubna Pal, Emre Seli, Speroff's Clinical Gynaecologic Endroclinology and Infertility, 9th Edition : 798.
4. Mauvais-Jarvis F, Manson JE, Stevenson JC, Fonseca VA. Menopausal Hormone Therapy and Type 2 Diabetes Prevention: Evidence, Mechanism and Clinical Implications. Endocr Rev. 2017;38(3):173-188.
5. Meeta Digmurti L, Vaze N et al., Clinical Practice Guidelines of Menopause, IMS, 2020.

6. Mueck AO, Seeger H. Effect of Hormone Therapy on BP in Normotensive and Hypertensive Post Menopausal Women. Maturitas. 2004;49(3):189-203.
7. N Aggarwal, B Shah, R Bansal ; Menopause Hormone Therapy in Comorbidies, Meeta's Clinical update on MHT (2024).
8. Stevenson JC. Best Practice & Research Clinical Obstetrics and Gynaecology 23 (2009):109–120.
9. The North American Menopause Society (NAMS) 2023 Guidelines.

CHAPTER 6

Hormone Replacement Therapy (HRT) in Women with Migraine Practical Decision Pathways

Renu Meena

INTRODUCTION

- Migraine is highly prevalent in women, particularly around reproductive age.
- Hormonal fluctuations play a major role in migraine pathophysiology.
- During perimenopause, unstable estrogen levels can worsen migraine frequency and severity.
- Postmenopause, migraine pattern may stabilize, but vasomotor symptoms (VMS)hot flashes, sleep disturbance, mood swings—may severely impact quality of life.
- HRT can be safely used in many migraine patients when prescribed thoughtfully, with individualized formulation, dose, and route.

TYPES OF MIGRAINE

Migraine Without Aura

- Recurrent throbbing headache with nausea, photophobia/phonophobia.
- Not associated with increased stroke risk if no other risk factors.

Migraine with Aura

- Neurological symptoms: visual, sensory or speech disturbances preceding headache.
- Associated with increased ischemic stroke risk, especially when combined with smoking or high estrogen states.

Perimenopausal Migraine

- Usually worsens due to fluctuating estrogen.
- Postmenopausal Migraine
- May improve due to estrogen stabilization.

Why Migraine Worsens During Perimenopause

- Estrogen levels fluctuate unpredictably in perimenopause → triggers migraine.
- Progesterone production becomes inconsistent → hormonal imbalance.

- Sleep disruption, anxiety, and vasomotor symptoms also decrease migraine threshold.

Why Consider HRT in Migraine Patients?

- To reduce vasomotor symptoms which themselves trigger migraines.
- To improve sleep quality, mood stability, and cognitive performance.
- To protect bone health and reduce risk of osteoporosis.
- To improve vulvovaginal atrophy, urinary symptoms, and sexual function.
- To improve overall quality of life.

BUT

- HRT is not used as a primary treatment of migraine, only to manage menopausal symptoms which subsequently reduce migraine frequency/severity.

Core Take-Home Principle

Migraine is not a contraindication to HRT.

What matters is:

- Type of migraine (with or without aura)
- Route of estrogen delivery
- Dose of estrogen
- Presence of vascular risk factors

Safety Considerations

- Migraine Without Aura→HRT is generally SAFE, especially with transdermal estrogen.
- Migraine With Aura → HRT can be used but requires:
- Lowest effective dose
- Transdermal route
- Avoid high-dose oral estrogen
- Optimize cardiovascular risk profile

Stroke and Vascular Risk – Clarification

- Migraine with aura alone: slightly increased stroke risk.
- Oral estrogen increases thrombotic risk → can compound stroke risk.
- Transdermal estrogen bypasses hepatic first-pass metabolism → minimal effect on clotting proteins → preferred route.

CONCLUSION

Use transdermal estradiol (patch/gel/spray) in all migraine patients needing HRT.

7 CHAPTER

MHT in Endometriosis

Jyoti Jaiswal

INTRODUCTION

MHT in Endometriosis

Endometriosis, an estrogen-dependent condition, often subsides with menopause. However, the onset of hypoestrogenism introduces new challenges—vasomotor symptoms, urogenital atrophy, and bone loss—leading many women to seek Hormone Replacement Therapy (HRT). Managing menopause in women with a history of endometriosis presents a unique challenge—how to relieve the distressing symptoms of estrogen deficiency without rekindling the dormant flames of the disease. Hormone Replacement Therapy (HRT) thus walks a fine line: offering relief, yet demanding caution. HRT in endometriosis must balance menopausal symptom relief with the risk of reactivation. Unopposed estrogen therapy is associated with recurrence and possible malignant transformation of residual lesions.

HRT in Menopausal and Postreproductive Age Group

As women transit into menopause, the need for hormonal support often arises. Following natural or surgical menopause, HRT is needed for symptom relief and osteoporosis prevention. Continuous combined estrogen-progestogen therapy or tibolone is recommended. Estrogen-only HRT should be avoided, even after hysterectomy, as it increases recurrence and malignancy risk. Transdermal estrogen with LNG-IUS is an effective alternative. Monitoring includes regular pelvic exams and imaging. Estradiol concentration that causes endometriosis lesions to grow or regress varies among women, but a concentration less than 20 pg/mL usually causes lesions to regress, and a concentration greater than 60 pg/mL usually supports lesion growth and maintains lesion viability. The estrogen threshold hypothesis suggests that gently suppressing estradiol to a concentration between 20 and 45 pg/mL may simultaneously cause endometriotic lesions to regress, resulting in reduced pelvic pain, minimal bone loss, and few hot flushes. Unopposed estrogen might carry the highest risk; therefore, the addition of progestogen would seem prudent, especially in extensive

TABLE 1: Age-wise Use of HRT in Endometriosis.

Age Group	*Purpose*	*Preferred Regimen*	*Precautions*
Prereproductive	Prevent hypoestrogenic effects during GnRH therapy	Add-back: Low-dose estrogen + progestin	Avoid excess estrogen
Reproductive	Suppress lesions, relieve pain	COC/Progestins/ GnRH + add-back	Avoid unopposed estrogen
Menopausal	Manage vasomotor and bone symptoms	Continuous combined HRT/ Tibolone	Monitor recurrence; avoid estrogen-only therapy

Flowchart 1: Decision Algorithm for HRT in Endometriosis.

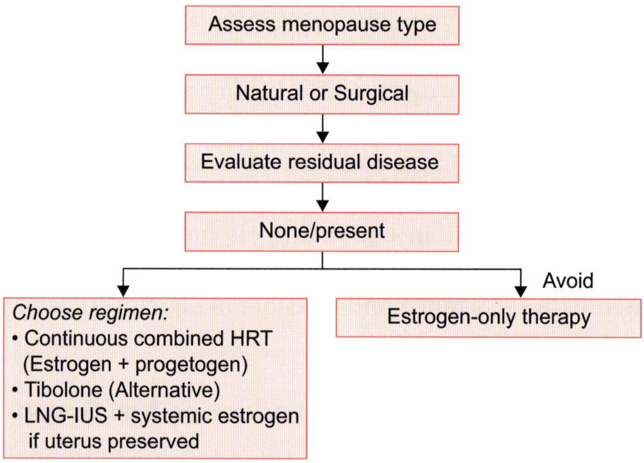

disease where surgery is deemed to be incomplete or in obese patients with higher levels of endogenous estrogens. The lowest effective dose is recommended. Avoid high doses. One can opt for additional nonhormonal options if needed.

KEY POINTS

- Endometriosis is an estrogen-dependent disease that can persist beyond menopause.
- HRT use must be individualized, balancing benefits and risks.
- Continuous combined HRT or tibolone are preferred regimens.
- Estrogen-only HRT is contraindicated even after hysterectomy.
- Add-back therapy is essential in younger women on GnRH analogues.
- Regular monitoring helps detect recurrence early.

TAKE-HOME MESSAGE

Relieve menopause—but don't rekindle endometriosis. HRT can safely be used in women with endometriosis if the regimen is appropriately selected. Continuous combined estrogen–progestogen therapy or tibolone or the lowest effective estrogen dose minimizes recurrence risk while improving quality of life. HRT must be individualized to aim for symptom control without stimulating residual disease—achieving *hormonal harmony with clinical vigilance.* Careful follow-up remains crucial for early detection of relapse or malignancy. The lowest effective dose is recommended. Avoid high doses. One can opt for additional nonhormonal options if needed.

SUGGESTED READING

1. Dave D, et al. Clinical management of endometriosis in menopause. Medicina. 2024;60(1):45–53.
2. Gemmell LC, et al. The management of menopause in women with a history of endometriosis. Hum Reprod Update. 2017;23(4):481–500.
3. Indian Menopause Society Clinical Practice Guidelines (2021).
4. Moghissi KS, et al. Zoladex with or without HRT in endometriosis. Fertil Steril. 1998;69(5):821–827.
5. Rosa-e-Silva JC, et al. Endometriosis in postmenopausal women without previous hormonal therapy. Climacteric. 2008;11(6):525–528.
6. Soliman NF, Hillard TC. Hormone replacement therapy in women with past history of endometriosis. Climacteric. 2006;9(5):325–335.
7. Streuli I, et al. Hormonal treatment of endometriosis: current options and perspectives. Int J Womens Health. 2013;5:597–611.
8. Vercellini P, et al. Endometriosis: pathogenesis and treatment. Nat Rev Endocrinol. 2014;10(5):261–275.

8 CHAPTER

Genitourinary Syndrome of Menopause Management

Kiran Aggarwal

GENITOURINARY SYNDROME OF MENOPAUSE

Menopause is a stage of life that is a physiological process encountered by all women. It is associated with depleting follicles in the ovaries and declining levels of estrogens in the body. Menopause is defined retrospectively when a woman has an amenorrhea of 12 months with loss of ovarian function for which no other pathology can be assigned.

GSM is estimated to affect between 27% and 84% of women in menopause.

It causes discomfort, sexual problems, deprivation of sleep and affects quality of life.

PATHOPHYSIOLOGY

- The genitourinary syndrome of menopause (GSM) is associated with menopause-related estrogen deficiency.
- This causes changes to the labia, vagina, urethra, and bladder and includes vulvovaginal atrophy.
- Lack of estrogens causes thinning of epithelium, loss of collagen, decreased elasticity and dryness.
- This causes vaginal irritation, pain, and atrophy, leading to dyspareunia and urinary tract problems.
- Lack of glycogen due to thinning of the epithelium leads to decreased acid production by lactobacillus and increased vaginal pH.
- In reproductive years vaginal mucosa has glycogen rich cells.
- The glycogen is changed by lactobacillus to lactic acid, and this keeps the vaginal pH between 3.5-4.5 and protects from infections.
- Due to a lack of estrogens in menopause, pH increases and vaginal atrophy occurs.

The symptoms are chronic and worsen with time. They adversely affect quality of life and need treatment.

Apart from natural menopause, Genitourinary syndrome of menopause may also be seen in primary ovarian insufficiency, use of antiestrogen drugs like Tamoxifen, aromatase inhibitors or after surgical menopause.

TERMINOLOGY

Previously, the condition was called as vulvovaginal atrophy or atrophic vaginitis. This did not address the urinary symptoms like recurrent Urinary tract infections and dysuria, etc. Therefore, this term was replaced in 2014 as Genitourinary syndrome of menopause by the International Society for the Study of Women's Sexual Health (ISSWSH) and the North American Menopause Society (NAMS) to describe the symptoms and signs associated with reduced levels of estrogens and androgens, leading to changes in the labia, clitoris, vestibule, introitus, vagina, urethra and bladder.

CLINICAL PRESENTATION

- A thorough history and detailed systemic and local examination are a must.
- The diagnosis of GSM is made when a woman presents with the following symptoms.
- Patient may present with vulval itching, pain, dryness, discomfort, dyspareunia, recurrent Urinary tract infections, urgency and frequency of urine.
- At times, vaginal discharge may be there.
- Any other pathology, like malignancy, infection, etc, should be ruled out.
- There may be decreased libido, postcoital bleeding, and it is associated with poor quality of life.
- The health care provider should ask for a targeted history, as the patient may be hesitant to respond

SIGNS ON CLINICAL EXAMINATION

- *Local:* Thinning of the labia majora, shrinking of the introitus.
- *On per speculum* examination, there may be pale vaginal mucosa without rugosities, loss of elasticity, a decrease in moisture, presence of petechiae.
- At times, infection and discharge may also be present. The cervix may be flushed with the vagina.
- *A vaginal health index* may be calculated to perform an objective assessment of the examination.
- It assesses *vaginal pH*.
- Loss of elasticity is marked by the absence of rugosities.
- Lack of fluid and moisture is seen, and the presence or absence of petechiae is noted.
- pH may be determined by placing a litmus paper in the side wall of the vagina for 30 seconds.
- If changes are more than 5, it signifies vaginal atrophy.
- A VHI less than 15 is indicative of vaginal atrophy.
- Vaginal maturation index may be calculated, but it is more of an academic exercise.

- Other conditions like lichen simplex chronicus, lichen planus, infections and malignancies should be ruled out.

INVESTIGATIONS

A hemogram, Blood sugar fasting, urine microscopy and culture should be done. Cervical cytology should be done.

MANAGEMENT OF GSM

The management of GSM should be need-based and depend on the symptoms. Comorbidities should be addressed.

LIFESTYLE, NUTRITION AND PHYSIOTHERAPY

The woman should be asked to maintain a healthy weight, do regular exercise. A sedentary lifestyle is associated with an increase in the prevalence of GSM. Regular supplementation of Vitamin D and calcium should be done. Alcohol and smoking should be avoided.

She should be counselled that sexual activity would improve blood flow to the vagina and will improve elasticity and moisture.

Comorbidities like Diabetes, hypertension, and dyslipidemias should be managed.

Pelvic floor muscle rehabilitation therapy can also be used along with other lifestyle management, like exercise, nutrition. Pelvic floor muscle exercises are taught. They improve tone and vascularity.

MOISTURIZERS AND LUBRICANTS

- Vaginal moisturizers are water-based with natural or synthetic polymers.
- They increase the moisture and improve the normal vaginal microbiome, and decrease pH.
- They decrease vaginal discomfort and dryness.
- Their effect lasts for two to three days, which is longer than that of lubricants.
- Hyaluronic-containing mosiutriseres are safe and effective.
- They should be used two times in a week.

Lubricants: They can be water, oil or silicone-based and is used before coitus.
- Their effect is short-lasting.

HORMONAL THERAPY

Local Estrogen Therapy

When lifestyle measurements and nonhormonal management fail or there are moderate to severe symptoms, local vaginal estrogens application is indicated.

Local estrogens improve vascularity, thickness of vaginal epithelium, improves pH and moisture.

Patient's symptoms improve, and also sexual function.

There is minimal absorption in the systemic circulation; therefore, progestogens are not indicated for endometrial protection.

PREPARATIONS

- Estradiol, conjugated equine estrogen and estriol are available to use vaginally.
- Low-dose estradiol (25 μg) and ultra-low-dose estradiol (4-10 μg) are effective.
- Low-dose conjugated equine estrogen cream (0.625 mg active ingredient/g/) and estriol (0.01% w/w) cream are the available formulations in India.

Dosage: They should be used daily for the initial two weeks, followed by alternate-day or twice a week application for 3- 6 months.

It may need a long treatment, but safety has been ascertained for one year of use.

Menopause Hormone Therapy (MHT): If oral hormonal therapy is being used for vasomotor symptoms, it will also alleviate GSM symptoms. However, in severe atrophy or symptoms, additional local therapy may be needed.

Dehydroepiandrosterone (DHEA): It is a precursor to sex hormones. When applied locally in the vagina, it gets converted to estrogen and androgens.

It improves vascularity and improves pH and moisture. It improves dryness and sexual function.

Daily dose is 6.5mg vaginally pessary daily. Discharge may be a side effect.

Ospemifene: It is the only oral therapy available for GSM. It is FDA approved. It can be used in treated cases of breast and endometrial cancers. Ospemifene is a Selective Estrogen Receptor Modulator (SERM). This means it acts like estrogen in some tissues but not in others. In vaginal tissues, ospemifene acts as an estrogen agonist, promoting tissue maturation and improving symptoms of Vulvovaginal Atrophy (VVA).

Energy-based devices: Lasers and radio frequency devices are being used, but none have been FDA-approved. They improve collagen synthesis, moisture is improved, and vascularization occurs.

CONCLUSION

- GSM is one of the symptoms of menopause. Most of the women are hesitant to complain and get themselves examined. The healthcare workers need to be educated about this condition. They should ask a detailed history with leading questions and assess clinically.

- Treatment with a trained professional and follow-up is important. Treatment helps improve symptoms and quality of life.
- Available estrogen creams for vagina in India
  - Evalon
  - Premarin

SUGGESTED READING

1. Briggs P, Hapangama DK. Urogenital atrophy: The 'unknown factors' challenging current practice. Post Reprod Health. 2021;27(2):109-120.
2. Cipriani S, Maseroli E, Ravelli SA, Vignozzi L. The vagina as source and target of androgens: implications for treatment of GSM/VVA, including DHEA. Vol. 26, Climacteric. Taylor and Francis Ltd.; 2023;p. 309-15.
3. Cox P, Panay N. Non-hormonal treatments for managing vulvovaginal atrophy/genitourinary syndrome of menopause. Vol. 26, Climacteric. Taylor and Francis Ltd.; 2023;p.367–72.
4. Da Silva AS, Baines G, Araklitis G, Robinson D, Cardozo L. Modern management of genitourinary syndrome of menopause. Fac Rev [Internet]. 2021 Mar 3;10. Available from: https://facultyopinions.com/prime/reports/b/10/25/
5. Faubion SS, Kingsberg SA, Clark AL, Kaunitz AM, Spadt SK, Larkin LC, et al. The 2020 genitourinary syndrome of menopause position statement of the North American Menopause Society. Menopause. 2020;27(9):976-92.
6. Kaufman MR, Lenore Ackerman A, Amin KA, Coffey M, Faubion SS, Hardart A, et al. Guideline Panel Staff and Consultants Systematic Review prepared by the Minnesota Evidence-based Practice Center Minneapolis, MN. Investigators. 2025.
7. Mercier J, Dumoulin C, Carrier-Noreau G. Pelvic floor muscle rehabilitation for genitourinary syndrome of menopause: why, how and when? Vol. 26, Climacteric. Taylor and Francis Ltd.; 2023;p.302-8.
8. Portman DJ, Gass MLS. Genitourinary syndrome of menopause: New terminology for vulvovaginal atrophy from the International Society for the Study of Women's Sexual Health and The North American Menopause Society. Climacteric. 2014;17(5):557-63.

9 CHAPTER

Tibolone

Ushma Maniar

INTRODUCTION

Tibolone was first developed in the 1960s and first tested for its effects on bone loss in the early 1970s. It was first introduced in the Netherlands in 1988 after nearly 25 years of extensive studies.

Pharmacokinetics

Tibolone is a synthetic estrane steroid. It is also known as 7α-methylnoretynodrel. It is a STEAR – Selective Tissue Estrogenic Activity Regulator – due to its regulation of estrogenic activity in a tissue-selective manner. It demonstrates estrogenic effects in tissues of the brain, bone, and vagina, while simultaneously avoiding the undesirable estrogenic effects on the breast and endometrium.

Tibolone has estrogenic, progestogenic and androgenic properties, and it demonstrates a unique metabolism as evidenced by different hormonal activities at different sites.

On oral administration, Tibolone is rapidly metabolized by the enzyme CYP2D6 into 3 biologically active metabolites:

- 3α – OH – tibolone – estrogenic activity
- 3β – OH – tibolone – estrogenic activity
- Δ4 isomer of Tibolone has progestogenic and androgenic activities

This conversion occurs mainly in the liver, and thus the excretion of Tibolone is mainly in the form of conjugated metabolites (sulphates).

INDICATIONS

- Post menopausal woman with Vasomotor Symptoms (VMS) affecting Quality of Life (QOL) (especially in those with low sex drive or FSD)
- Mood disorders and women receiving psychoactive treatment
- Vaginal dryness
- Osteopenic and osteoporotic PMW
- Premature menopause and POI
- Surgical menopause (especially for endometriosis and in those with BSO
- Women with breast tenderness, mastalgia and fibroadenosis
- Women with mammographically dense breasts

- PMW with co-existing uterine factors (especially fibroids, endometriosis and adenomyosis)
- PMW suffering from Genito Urinary Syndrome of Menopause (GUSM)
- Women who receive long term add back Gonadotrophic Releasing Hormone (GnRH) agonists - The unique structure of Tibolone helps prevent bone loss in these patients.

CONTRAINDICATIONS

Absolute	*Relative*
Undiagnosed vaginal bleeding	Age > 60 years or >10 years from FMP
Pregnancy or suspected pregnancy	Gall bladder diseases
Current or prior endometrial cancer	Smoking
Breast cancers	Migraine
Established CVD or those with an increased risk of stroke	Moderate risk of CVD
Arterial thromboembolism Example – Angina, MI, TIA	Past history of DVT or Varicose Vein
Personal or family history of VTE	
Known thrombophilia and porphyria	
Morbid obesity	
Diabetes with end-organ disease	
Systemic Lupus Erythematosus (SLE)	
Severe active liver disease and impaired LFT	

DOSAGE AND PRESCRIPTIONS

Tibolone is to be prescribed at a dosage of 1.25 or 2.5 g/day, preferably same time daily and without a break.

Before starting therapy, a detailed history including symptoms, Final Menstrual Period (FMP), personal and family history, addictions, allergies, thorough clinical examination including BMI, BP, CVS and CNS examination, local examination, PS, TVS and blood investigations, including LFT should be done.

Tibolone can be started immediately after surgical menopause.

Tibolone should be started one year after natural menopause due to the risk of occasional irregular vaginal bleeding or spotting.

When switching over from MHT or OCP, it is advisable to wait for a withdrawal bleed as the endometrium may already be stimulated.

The patient needs to be counselled that the effects will be visible after 3 to 4 weeks and has to be continued for 3 months minimum to have a satisfactory response.

The duration of the treatment has to be individualized. It is reasonably safe to prescribe Tibolone for long durations, uninterrupted. However, it is NOT advisable to continue beyond 65 years of age.

Follow-Up

- 1 month - for side effects and adherence.
- 3 months, 6 months, Anually - for effectiveness, side effects and investigations.

Side Effects

- Nausea
- *Bleeding:* Occasionally, random bleeding episodes have been reported within the first three to four months of usage. It stops spontaneously. In extremely rare cases, bleeding can occur after six months. In this case, the bleeding has to be thoroughly evaluated as a case of post-menopausal bleeding.
- *Weight Gain*
- *Breast Tenderness.*
- *Androgenic Effects* – facial hair growth and abdominal fat collection.

Drug Interactions

- *WARFARIN:* Tibolone increases fibrinolytic activity, so contraindicated.
- *Enzyme Inducers:* They reduce the serum level of Tibolone.
- *Insulin and OHAs:* Tibolone has a favorable effect on the sugar profile and increases insulin sensitivity in the body.
- *Hepatotoxic Drugs:* Tibolone is extensively metabolized in the liver. Hence, hepatotoxic drugs are absolutely contraindicated with Tibolone use.
- *Oral Estrogens:* It is not recommended to simultaneously prescribe estrogens with Tibolone as it can cause vaginal bleeding.
- *Paroxetine:* Paroxetine inhibits the CYP2D6 enzyme, which is required for the metabolism of Tibolone. Hence, Paroxetine cannot be co-administered with Tibolone.

Systemic Effects of Tibolone

Sexuality

MoA: The Δ4 isomer reduces SHBG, and thus increases bioavailable testosterone, estradiol (E_2) and dehydroepiandrosterone sulphate (DHEA-s). the androgenic effect improves libido. The overall effect is an increase in sexual interest, fantasies, arousal and orgasm.

The Livial International Study in Sexual Arousal (LISA) concluded that Tibolone significantly relieves climacteric symptoms and improves mood and well-being.

The Tolerability Trial (TOTAL) study showed an improvement in vaginal atrophy, maturation index and karyopyknotic index in the vaginal epithelium, compared to conventional MHT. These combined effects cause improved mood, libido and sexual excitement.

Bone

MoA: Tibolone has an estrogenic effect on bone, thus inhibiting bone resorption by reducing osteoclastic activity. Tibolone reduces the incidence of BOTH, vertebral and non-vertebral fractures.

Long Term Intervention on Fractures with Tibolone (LIFT) study. When compared to placebo, Tibolone decreases the relative hazards of osteoporosis related vertebral and non-vertebral fractures. However, in elderly women, Tibolone increase the chance of stoke. Hence, it is best avoided in women >70 years.

The Tibolone Histology of the Endometrium and Breast End Points Study (THEBES) showed reduction of fracture in younger women (mean age 55 years).

Osteoporosis Prevention and Arterial Effects (OPAL) study concluded that Tibolone increases BMD and reduces fracture risk, similar to estrogen therapy.

VMS

MoA: Tibolone is rapidly metabolized to active estrogen metabolites, which replace the diminishing estrogen levels in effect regulating the body's temperature control and thus hot flushes.

Neuropsychiatric Symptoms

MoA: Tibolone increases β endorphin and β lipoprotein levels, thus improving mood and relieving insomnia. This effect is more pronounced in Asian women.

QOL

MoA: Tibolone increases allopregnanolone, a steroid with sedative and anxiolytic properties. At the same time, it does not reduce adrenal function in menopause, making it a superior drug compared to estrogen.

Uterus

MoA: The Δ isomer binds to progesterone receptor and protects the endometrium against the estrogenic metabolites.

Fibroids: There is no evidence of myoma growth on women taking Tibolone. In fact, add back therapy with Tibolone prevents flushing and bone loss in those treated with GnRH.

Breast

MoA: In breast tissue, Tibolone inhibits sulfatase activity effectively, blocking the conversion of estrone sulphate to estrone, thus acting like a progestin and weak androgen in the breast. Thus, it increases cell differentiation and stimulates apoptosis. The overall effect is a reduction in the risk of breast carcinoma.

LIFT trial showed that Tibolone group had a decreased risk of invasive breast and colon cancer.

Livial Intervention following Breast Carcinoma (LIBERATE) trial concluded that Tibolone increases the chances of recurrent breast carcinoma in those with a past history of ER positive breast carcinoma.

CVS

MoA: Tibolone decreases:

- Total cholesterol
- LDL
- Triglycerides
- Lipoprotein A
- HDL

Tibolone activates the nitrous oxide production via estrogenic effects. Hence it also has a lipid independent cardioprotective expression in the endothelial cells.

OPAL study revealed that Tibolone has complex effects on cardiovascular risk factors, including lowering HDL cholesterol and was less favorable on CVS, compared to EPT.

Venous Thromboembolism (VTE) and Stroke

MoA: Tibolone decreases the fibrinogen and factor VII activity and increases antithrombin III and plasminogen activity so the net effect is an increase in fibrinolytic activity. Tibolone has no effect on hypertension.

LIFT study showed a neutral effect of Tibolone on coagulation, but a 2 times increase in risk of stroke in women >70 years of age.

Diabetes

- Tibolone increases insulin sensitivity in woman with insulin resistance.
- Tibolone can safely be used in women with well controlled diabetes and HTN.

Research

CCDC114, DNAI2 and TOP2A genes are involved in the effect of Tibolone on endometrium.

KEY POINTS

- Tibolone is approved for use in 90 countries in Asia and Europe for menopausal symptoms and in 45 countries to prevent osteoporosis, but it is not FDA-approved in the USA.
- It is a STEAR with excellent tissue-specific actions with estrogenic effect on bone, brain and vagina and antiestrogenic effect on breast and endometrium.
- It is the preferred drug in PMW, where VMS and FSD co-exist.
- It reduces the risk of both vertebral and non-vertebral fractures in osteoporotic women and is more effective than Raloxifen for the same.
- It is preferable over MHT in women with mammographically dense breasts.
- It can be given to PMW with well controlled diabetes and hypertension.
- A lot of research with Tibolone, especially in Indian scenario, needs to be done before its general and widespread use.

SUGGESTED READING

1. Anil Sadarangani, Ana Maria et al. In vivo and in vitro estrogenic and progestogenic actions of Tibolone. Biol Res. 2005;38(2-3):245-258.
2. Bhattacharya SM. Effects of Tibolone on health related quality of life in menopausal women. Int. J. Gynobs. 2007;99(1):43-45.
3. Bots ML, Evans GW, Riley W et al. The effect of Tibolone and continuous CEE plus MPA on progression of carotid intima media thickness; OPAL study. Eur Heart J. 2006;27(6)746-755.
4. Cummings SR, Ettinger B, Delmas PD, et al. The effects of Tibolone in older PMW. N Engl J Med. 2008;359(7):697-708.
5. David F. Archer et al THEBES. Fertil Steril. 2007 Oct;88(4):866-878.
6. Erel CT, Elter K, Akman C, et al. Mammographic changes in women receiving tibolone therapy. Fertil Steril. 1998;69(5):870-5.
7. Formoso G, Perrone E, Maltoni S, et al. Short-term and long-term effects of Tibolone in PMW. Cochrane Database Syst Rev. 2016;10(10):CD008536.
8. Genazzani AR, Pluchino N, Bernardi F, Centofanti M, Luisi M. Beneficial effect of Tibolone on mood cognition, well-being and sexuality in menopausal women. Neuropsychiatr Dis Treat. 2006;2(3):299-307
9. Huang KE, Baber R; Asia Pacific Tibolone Consensus Group. Updated clinical recommendations for use of Tibolone in Asian women. Climacteric. 2010;13(4):317-27.
10. Hudita D, Posea C, Ceausu I, Rusu M. Efficacy and safety of oral tibolone 1.25 or 2.5 mg/day vs. placebo in postmenopausal women. Eur Rev Med Pharmacol Sci. 2003;7(5):117-25.
11. Koh KK, Ahn JY et al. Significant differential effects of hormone therapy or Tibolone on markers of CVS disease in PMW. Arterioscl. Thromb. Vasc Bio 2003;23(10):1889-94.

12. Laan E, van Lunsen RH, Everaerd W. The effects of Tibolone on vaginal blood flow, sexual desire and arousability in PMW. Climacteric. 2001;4(1):28-41.
13. Malik R, Meghana Reddy P. Effectiveness of Tibolone in relieving post-menopausal symptoms for a short-term period in Indian women. JOGI. J Obstet Gynaecol India. 2023;73(3):242-247.
14. Morris EP, Rymer J, Robinson J, Fogelman I. Efficacy of Tibolone as Add-back therapy in conjunction with GnRH analogue in treatment of fibroids. Fertil Steril. 2008;89(2):421-8.
15. Somunkiran A, Erel CT, Demirci F, Senturk ML. The effect of tibolone versus 17beta-estradiol on climacteric symptoms in women with surgical menopause: a randomized, cross-over study. Maturitas. 2007;56(1):61-8.
16. Yanhua LV, Yanqing Liu, Yeuqiang. CCDC114, DNAI2, TOP2A involved in the effect of Tibolone on the endometrium. BMC Women's Health. 2021;21:240.

10 CHAPTER

Adult Vaccination: What's Important, What's Essential

Meenakshi Ahuja, Aarshika Singh

INTRODUCTION

Vaccination is widely recognized as a pillar of preventive health. While most immunization programes focus on childhood, adult vaccination (particularly in the mid-life/40-65 age-group) is increasingly important due to age-related decline in immunity, comorbidities and changing lifestyles. In India, although much attention is given to childhood vaccination, adult immunization remains an under-recognized domain. The global agencies, such as the World Health Organization (WHO) emphasise life-course immunization, and national bodies such as the Indian Council of Medical Research (ICMR), together with the Ministry of Health and Family Welfare (MoHFW) need to advance adult-vaccination policies. The Centres for Disease Control and Prevention (CDC) in the United States has long maintained adult immunization schedules which provide a useful model. This article summarizes current international and Indian guidelines, outlines key vaccine-preventable diseases (VPDs) in adults, and gives practical recommendations for mid-life workshops.

GUIDING FRAMEWORKS AND RECOMMENDATIONS

- *WHO:* The WHO "Recommendations for routine immunization - summary tables" include immunization across the life-course, emphasizing that adults receive appropriate booster doses and catch-up immunization.
- *CDC:* The CDC publishes an "Adult Immunization Schedule by Age (19 years or older)" which covers recommended vaccines for adults.
- India (ICMR/MoHFW): In India, adult immunization guidelines are less fully integrated into national policy. The ICMR/MoHFW, through the National Centre for Disease Control (NCDC) have published an adult immunization document, noting the sizable burden of adult VPDs and the need for adult vaccination.
- *Indian Consensus Guidelines:* The Association of Physicians of India (API) has produced a consensus guideline on adult immunization in India, which consolidates international guidance and adapts to the Indian context.
- *Implementation context:* Reviews of the Indian situation highlight that although adult vaccination is recognized, uptake remains low, awareness

is poor, and national vaccination policy still focuses mainly on childhood and pregnancy.

Key Vaccine-Preventable Diseases (VPDs) in Adults & Recommended Vaccines

Below is a summary of selected VPDs relevant to mid-life adults in India. For each disease: definition and relevance, Indian guideline summary, and practical points.

Influenza

Definition/relevance: Influenza is an acute viral respiratory infection which in adults can lead to severe illness, hospitalization, exacerbation of chronic diseases and death. In older adults and those with comorbidities, the risk is high.

Guideline summary: In India, adult influenza vaccination (especially for those aged >50 years or with chronic diseases) is recommended by expert consensus. The CDC recommends annual influenza vaccination for all adults.

Practical points: In a mid-life workshop, emphasize annual influenza vaccination before the influenza season, especially for those with diabetes, cardiovascular or lung disease, and encourage uptake in working adults and caregivers.

Pneumococcal Disease (e.g., Pneumonia, Invasive Pneumococcal Disease)

Definition/relevance: Pneumococcal disease caused by Streptococcus pneumoniae is a major cause of community-acquired pneumonia, sepsis and meningitis, especially in adults >65 years and those with chronic conditions.

Guideline summary: Indian guideline reviews suggest pneumococcal vaccination for healthy adults >65 years and for younger adults with risk factors. The CDC schedule similarly recommends pneumococcal vaccines for adults ≥65 years and younger adults at risk.

Practical points: In mid-life, screen for risk factors (e.g., COPD, heart disease, diabetes, smoking) and offer pneumococcal vaccine as appropriate. Also use as an opportunity to counsel on smoking cessation, lung health and immunization. PCV (Pneumococcal Conjugate Vaccine) and PPSV23 (Pneumococcal Polysaccharide Vaccine) are available in India.

Tetanus/Diphtheria/Pertussis (Td/Tdap)

Definition/relevance: Tetanus, diphtheria and pertussis remain vaccine-preventable infections; adult boosters are required to maintain immunity. Especially pertussis in adults may transmit to infants.

Guideline summary: Indian guidelines indicate that for adults ≥18 years who have completed childhood primary vaccination, a Td booster every 10 years up to age 65 is indicated; one dose of Tdap may be substituted for Td in certain circumstances (e.g., contact with infants). CDC recommends one dose of Tdap and then Td or Tdap every 10 years.

Practical points: Emphasize to mid-life participants the need for adult boosters even if childhood vaccination was given, and highlight special roles (e.g., pregnancy, contact with infants, health-care workers).

Hepatitis B

Definition/relevance: Hepatitis B virus infection can lead to chronic liver disease and hepatocellular carcinoma; adults at risk include those with occupational exposure, comorbid liver disease, diabetes, multiple sexual partners, or travel.

Guideline summary: While India's childhood hepatitis B immunization is well-established, adult vaccination is recommended for risk groups by consensus. The CDC recommends hepatitis B vaccination for adults ages 19–59 and older adults with risk factors.

Practical points: In mid-life workshops, screen for hepatitis B risk factors, and encourage vaccination for those unvaccinated, with focus on lifestyle risk, comorbidities (e.g., diabetes) and family-history of liver disease.

Herpes Zoster (Shingles)

Definition/relevance: Herpes zoster is the reactivation of varicella (chickenpox) virus in adults, more likely in older age and in those with declining immunity; it can cause painful and debilitating complications (post-herpetic neuralgia).

Guideline summary: Indian guideline reviews suggest zoster vaccine for adults >60 years. The WHO and other international bodies support zoster vaccination in older adults.

Practical points: In mid-life workshops (ages ~50+), introduce the concept of shingles vaccine, discuss risk reduction, and guide participants towards discussing vaccination with their physician, especially if they have underlying immunosuppression or chronic disease.

Shingrix (GSK) 2 doses 6 months apart

Human Papillomavirus (HPV)

Definition/relevance: The Human papillomavirus infection causes genital warts, precancerous lesions and cancers (cervical, oropharyngeal, anal). While widely promoted in adolescents, catch-up in young adults may be beneficial.

Guideline summary: Indian consensus guidelines include HPV vaccination for healthy adults in defined age groups. CDC recommends HPV vaccination through age 26, and some adults ages 27-45 based on shared decision-making.

Practical points: In a mid-life workshop (especially inclusive of younger mid-life, say 30–45 years), highlight HPV vaccination as an adult preventive measure when not done earlier, and integrate this into a broader preventive health conversation (cancers, screening, lifestyle).

IMPLEMENTATION AND PRACTICAL WORKSHOP POINTS

- *Use a life-course approach:* Emphasize that immunization is not only for childhood, but extends into adulthood and older age.
- *Conduct risk-screening in the workshop:* Age, comorbidities (diabetes, heart disease, COPD, liver disease), occupational risk, lifestyle (smoking, travel), prior vaccination history.
- *Provide clear tables/flowcharts:* E.g., "Which vaccines do I need now (ages 40–65)?" "Booster schedule for tetanus/diphtheria/pertussis" etc.
- *Address barriers:* Low awareness among adults, vaccine hesitancy, cost issues, absence of adult immunization programes in many settings in India.
- *Encourage linkage with health-care providers:* Adults should be advised to discuss with their physicians, check vaccination records, check for comorbidities and receive appropriate vaccines.

TABLE 1: Summary of Adult Vaccines and Indications.

Vaccine	*Indication/age group*	*Key reminders*
Influenza	All adults annually, especially >50 or with comorbidities	Annual dose, before flu season
Pneumococcal	Adults >65 years, or younger with risk (diabetes, lung, heart diseases)	Check risk status, one-time or sequential dosing as per schedule
Td/Tdap Tetanus/ diphtheria	Adults every 10 years (or one Tdap then Td/Tdap booster)	Especially healthcare workers, pregnant women, contact with infants
Hepatitis B	Adults with risk factors (liver disease, diabetes, occupational exposure)	Complete series if not done earlier
Herpes zoster (shingles)	Adults >=60 years (or earlier if risk)	Two-dose schedule for eligible adults
HPV (Human papilloma virus)	Adults up to age ~45 years who were not vaccinated earlier	Shared decision-making, especially in younger mid-life

- *Integrate with broader preventive health:* While focusing on immunization, link with other mid-life health checks (e.g., blood pressure, cholesterol, diabetes, cancer screening) to enhance the "wellness" message.
- *Use take-home resources:* Provide hand-outs or checklists for participants to take to their physician, e.g., "Adult Immunization Checklist".

KEY POINTS (TAKE-HOME MESSAGES)

Adult vaccination is a vital, yet under-utilized, component of preventive health in the mid-life population. A life-course approach to immunization means that adults aged 40-65 should review their vaccination status, especially in the presence of chronic diseases, lifestyle risk factors or occupational exposures. Key vaccines in the Indian context include influenza (annually), pneumococcal (especially if ≥65 or with risk), Td/Tdap boosters every 10 years, hepatitis B (for risk-groups), herpes zoster (for older adults), and HPV (when not given earlier). International guidelines from WHO, CDC and Indian consensus recommend clear schedules and indications. The challenge in India remains low adult-vaccine awareness and lack of routine adult-immunization policy. Workshops like this should empower individuals to ask their physicians about adult vaccines, integrate immunization into broader mid-life health planning, and use simple tools (checklists, screening forms) to bridge the gap between awareness and action.

SUGGESTED READING

1. Association of Physicians of India. Indian Consensus Guideline on Adult Immunization. API; 2024.
2. Centers for Disease Control and Prevention. Adult Immunization Schedule by Age – United States, 2025. [Internet] 2025. Available from: https://www.cdc.gov/vaccines/hcp/imz-schedules/adult-age.html
3. Centers for Disease Control and Prevention. Immunization Schedules | Vaccines & Immunizations. [Internet] 2025. Available from: https://www.cdc.gov/vaccines/hcp/imz-schedules/index.html
4. Dhawan AM, Desai A, Gvalani A, Anand S, Das P. A comprehensive review of the recent adult immunization guidelines by the Association of Physicians of India. Int J Community Med Public Health. 2025;12(2):1159-1165.
5. Garg S, Dey AK, Tripathy JP et al. Towards adult vaccination in India: a narrative literature review. J Fam Med Prim Care. 2022;11(8):3575-3581.
6. Gupta S, et al. Guidelines for vaccination in normal adults in India. Indian J Community Med. 2016;41(3):??.
7. Jain A, Sharma P, et al. Adult vaccination in India: A rapid review of current status, implementation challenges. Indian J Med Res. 2024;149(3):XX-XX.
8. Mayo Clinic. Vaccines for adults: Which do I need? Mayo Clinic. 2024. Available from: https://www.mayoclinic.org/healthy-lifestyle/adult-health/in-depth/vaccines/art-20046750
9. NCDC/MoHFW. Adult Immunization – CD Alert. New Delhi: Government of India; 2024.
10. World Health Organization. WHO recommendations for routine immunization—summary tables. [Internet] 2024. Available from: https://www.who.int/teams/immunization-vaccines-and-biologicals/policies/who-recommendations-for-routine-immunization

11 CHAPTER

Menopausal Symptoms, Menopause Risk and Their Assessment

Renuka Malik

The women in menopause and the transition phase experience symptoms and are unprepared for it. The clinician should be aware of these symptoms and method to assess them. The symptoms experienced by women include:

1. *Vasomotor symptoms:* Hot flashes and night sweats
2. *Mood changes:* irritability, anxiety, depression
3. *Vaginal dryness* and discomfort during intercourse
4. Sleep disturbances and fatigue
5. Weight gain or changes in body composition
6. Body aches and pain
7. Memory issues or 'brain fog'

THE SUBJECTIVE QUESTIONNAIRES FOR MENOPAUSAL SYMPTOMS

Menopause Rating Score Questionnaire (MRS)

Which of the following symptoms apply to you at this time?

Assessment

The postmenopausal symptoms were graded according to the severity. MRS consists of a list of 11 symptoms which are divided into 3 subscales- *Somatic subscale* (Hot flashes, heart discomfort, sleep disorder, joint and muscular discomfort) corresponding to questions 1, 2, 3 and 11 respectively, *Psychological subscale* (Depressive mood, irritability, anxiety, physical and mental exhaustion) corresponding to questions 4, 5, 6 and 7 respectively and *Urogenital subscale* (Sexual problems, bladder problems, dryness of vagina). corresponding to questions 8, 9 and 10 respectively. Patients graded their symptoms in a 5 point (0-4) likert scale as none (0) mild (1), moderate (2), severe (3)and very severe as 4 **(Table 1)**. Score were added and individual sub scale and total menopausal score calculated and graded. The Total score varied from 0 to 44.

0-4 is graded as none or minimal menopausal symptoms

5- 8 as mild menopausal symptoms,

9-15 as moderate and

16-44 as severe post menopausal symptoms.

TABLE 1: Menopause rating questionnaire.

(X ONE Box For EACH Symptom) *For Symptoms That Do Not Apply, Please Mark "None")*						
Symptoms:		***None***	***Mild***	***Moderate***	***Severe***	***Extremely Severe***
	Score =	***0***	***1***	***2***	***3***	***4***
1.	Hot flashes, sweating (episodes of sweating)	☐	☐	☐	☐	☐
2.	Heart discomfort (unusual awareness of heart beat, heart skipping, heart racing, tightness)	☐	☐	☐	☐	☐
3.	Sleep problems (difficulty in falling asleep, difficulty in sleeping through the night, waking up early)	☐	☐	☐	☐	☐
4.	Depressive mood (feeling down, sad, on the verge of tears, lack of drive, mood swings).	☐	☐	☐	☐	☐
5.	Irritability (feeling nervous, inner tension, feeling aggressive)	☐	☐	☐	☐	☐
6.	Anxiety (inner restlessness, feeling panicky)	☐	☐	☐	☐	☐
7.	Physical and mental exhaustion (general decrease in performance, impaired memory, decrease in concentration, forgetfulness).	☐	☐	☐	☐	☐
8.	Sexual problems (change in sexual desire, in sexual activity and satisfaction)	☐	☐	☐	☐	☐
9.	Bladder problems (difficulty in urinating, increased need to urinate, bladder incontinence).	☐	☐	☐	☐	☐
10.	Dryness of vagina (sensation of dryness or burning in the vagina, difficulty with sexual intercourse)	☐	☐	☐	☐	☐
11.	Joint and muscular discomfort (pain in the joints, rheumatoid complaints)	☐	☐	☐	☐	☐

The Greene Climacteric Scale

It consists of 21 items in four domains plus one sexual function probe. Greene Climacteric Scale consists of 21 questions covering 5 domains: anxiety, depression, somatic symptoms, vasomotor symptoms, and sexual function. Each question is answered on a 4-point Likert scale. The answers to all 21 questions are summed to give a total quality-of-life measure; a higher score indicates a worse quality of life.

GENITOURINARY SYNDROME OF MENOPAUSE

Vaginal pH Measurement

The most frequently used is the vaginal pH measurement, recommended since 2003 by the FDA for GSM assessment, and used as a part of the VHI calculation. To assess pH, a piece of litmus paper is placed on the lateral vaginal wall until moistened. A pH of 4.6 or greater indicates vulvovaginal atrophy (VVA), assuming the patient does not have bacterial vaginosis.

Vaginal Maturation Index

Another recommended outcome, in the 2003 FDA recommendation to GSM evaluation was the VMI, which has not been as successful in the literature as the VHI, considering that it is not usually found in most studies assessing GSM. Smear is made from middle lateral vaginal wall ,100 cells counted .The VMI assesses the relative proportion of parabasal(P), intermediate(I), and superficial vaginal epithelial cell (S)types in a vaginal cytology sample. In premenopausal women, greater than 15% of superficial cells would be considered normal. However, in postmenopausal women with VVA, the typical proportion would be less than 5%. The VMI is usually calculated according to the formula, maturation value: (0 × % of parabasal cells) + (0.5 × % of intermediate cells) +(1.0 × % of superficial cells).Another formula which is used is Another formula used is (0.2 × % P + 0.6 × % I + 1 × % S)

Vaginal Health Index

TABLE 2: Vaginal Health Index.

Score	*Overall elasticity*	*Type of fluid secretion & consistency*	*Vaginal pH*	*Vaginal epithelial mucosa*	*Moisture*
1	NONE	None	6.1	Petechiae noted before contact	None, inflamed mucosa
2	POOR (Scanty)	Thin yellow	5.6-6.0	Bleeds with light touch	None, mucosa not inflamed
3	FAIR (Superficial)	Thin white	5.1-5.5	Bleeds with scraping	Minimal
4	GOOD (Moderate)	Thin white	4.7-5.0	Not friable, thin mucosa	Moderate
5	EXCELLENT	Normal white flocculent	<=4.6	Not friable, normal mucosa	Normal

Less than 15 indicates vaginal atrophy.

METHODS TO ASSESS BONE AND MUSCLE HEALTH

- *Osteopenia/porosis* - BMD assessment by DEXA SCAN is the most widely used test. T score of less or equal to than -2.5 is taken as osteoporosis.
- *FRAX SCORE* with or without BMD is used as a screening tool. Other questionnaires like GARVAN, OST, and SCORE are also used. FRAX is a computer-based equation that uses clinical risk factors to estimate a patient's 10-year fracture probability. Although it has been validated in the general population, it has some limitations that may cause it to underestimate the fracture risk in postmenopausal women.
- *FRAX score*- The National Osteoporosis Foundation (NOF) ,now known as Bone Health and Osteoporosis Foundation (BHOF)] guidelines recommend initiation of treatment in patients with hip or vertebral fractures, patients whose T-score is in the osteoporotic range at the femoral neck, total hip or lumbar spine as assessed by DEXA, and in postmenopausal women and men older than 50 years with osteopenia and a 10-year major osteoporosis fracture probability assessed by the appropriate FRAX tool of ≥20% or a hip fracture probability ≥3%
- *FRAX* uses seven readily available dichotomous clinical risk factors (inserted as yes or no into the calculator): prior fragility fracture, parental hip fracture, smoking, systemic glucocorticoid use, excess alcohol intake, rheumatoid arthritis, and other causes of secondary osteoporosis. Other factors included in FRAX are age, sex, and body mass index (BMI). FRAX can calculate fracture probability with or without femoral neck BMD so accommodating situations where densitometric assessment is not available.

TABLE 3: Who Classification of postmenopausal osteoporosis

Classification	*T -Score (Sd)*
Normal	Equal to –1.0 or higher
Osteopenia (low bone mass)	Between –1.0 and 2.5
Osteoporosis	Equal to –2.5 or lower
Severe osteoporosis	Equal to –2.5 or lower with fracture

WHO Technical Report series 843.1994

SARCOPENIA ASSESSMENT

Subjective questionnaires like SARC F which is a self-administered, five item questionnaire on strength, assistance walking, rising from a chair, climbing stairs and falls. SARC-F score is given for each as 0, 1 or 2 with 4 as cut off. 4 or more score is a positive screening test for sarcopenia AWGS has added measurement of calf circumference to SARC. (SARC-CC) If calf circumference is less than 34 cm,(33 as per Asian cut of for Asian women)

10 points are added to SARC score. A score of 11 or more is taken as positive screening for sarcopenia.

SARC-F Screen for Sarcopenia: Component Question Scoring

Strength: How much difficulty do you have in lifting and carrying 10 pounds?

- None 0
- Some 1
- A lot or unable 2

Assistance in walking: How much difficulty do you have walking across a room?

- None 0
- Some 1
- A lot, use aids, or unable 2

Rise from a chair: How much difficulty do you have transferring from a chair or bed?

- None 0
- Some 1
- A lot or unable without help 2

Climb Stairs: How much difficulty do you have climbing a flight of 10 stairs?

- None 0
- Some 1
- A lot or unable 2

Falls: How many times have you fallen in the past year?

- None 0
- less than 3 falls 1
- 4 or more falls 2

Muscle Mass: The gold standard for measuring muscle mass is DEXA SCAN. MRI, CT scan, and Bio-impedance are other methods with lower sensitivity. Appendicular skeletal muscle index (ASMI), is a measure of muscle mass which is calculated by DEXA scan. Ultrasound also has low sensitivity. Calf muscle circumference can be used in community settings to assess sarcopenia. The cutoff point for low muscle mass of calf circumference for menopausal women was taken as <33 cm, according to the AWGS 2019.

Muscle Strength: it can be measured by hand held dynamometer. AWGS 2019 recommends low muscle strength diagnostic cutoffs of handgrip <18 kg for women.

Muscle performance can be measured by 4m gait test, timed up and go test (TUGT) and, chair stand test which are of two types-5-time chair stand test and one recommended by CDC.

5-Time chair stand test: The five-time chair-stand test ≥12 seconds indicates poor muscle performance and greater than 10 seconds showed an increased risk of disability onset, and greater than 13.7 seconds was associated with increased disability and morbidity.

Chair stand below average scores (CDC): Count the number of times the patient comes to a full standing position in 30 seconds. SCORING 60-64 years <12, 65-69 years <11, 70-74 years <10, 75-79 years <10, 80-84 years <9, 85-89 years <8, 90-94 years < 4.

BREAST CANCER AND CARDIAC RISK SCORE

Breast Cancer: Gail model and Tyrer-Cuzick model are commonly used.

1. *The breast cancer risk assessment tool (BCRAT)* also known as The Gail Model, allows health professionals to estimate a woman's risk of developing invasive breast cancer over the next five years and up to age 90 (lifetime risk). The tool uses a woman's personal medical and reproductive history and the history of breast cancer among her first-degree relatives (mother, sisters, daughters) to estimate absolute breast cancer risk-her chance or probability of developing invasive breast cancer in a defined age interval.
   This calculator takes about five minutes to complete.

   The tool uses a woman's own personal information to estimate risk of developing invasive breast cancer over specific periods of time, including:
   - Age
   - Age at the start of menstruation
   - Age at first live birth of a child
   - Number of first-degree relative (mother, sisters, daughters) with breast cancer
   - Number of previous breast biopsies (whether positive or negative)
   - Presence of atypical hyperplasia in a biopsy
2. *Tyrer-cuzick breast cancer risk model:* It is also as an online tool and takes father's breast cancer history into consideration too.

Cardiac Risk Calculators

They are available as online tools.

1. ASCVD RISK Alogithm: It determines 10-year risk of hard ASCVD,(atherosclerotic Cardiovascular disease)i.e. myocardial infarction, stroke, or death due to coronary heart disease or stroke, and provides statin recommendations. s calculator is for use only in adult patients without known ASCVD and LDL 70-189 mg/dL (1.81-4.90 mmol/L). The following parameters are recorded to get the risk assessment-Age (this calculator only applies to individuals 40-75 years of age.), diabetes, sex, smoker, total cholesterol, systolic blood pressure, treatment for hypertension and race.

2. *PREVENT score:* The PREVENT calculator, based on the PREVENT equations, uses required clinical information to estimate CVD risk. Three optional predictors, urine albumin-creatinine ratio (UACR), hemoglobin A1c (HbA1c), and social deprivation index (SDI), can further personalize risk estimates.

The PREVENT calculator provide separate 10-year and 30-year estimates for total CVD (PREVENT-CVD), ASCVD (PREVENT-ASCVD), and HF (PREVENT-HF).

MENTAL HEALTH

In addition women in perimenopause and menopause should also be screened for mental health in the form of asking for stress, depression and anxiety as they are independent risk factors

Sleep and Cognitive Function

Metabolic Syndrome: Diagnosed to have MetS, using NCEP ATP III criteria, if they had any three or more of the following: 1. Central obesity: Waist circumference ≥80 cm (south-Asian cutoff). 2. Hypertriglyceridemia: Serum TG level ≥ 150 mg/dL. 3. Low HDL cholesterol 4. High blood pressure: SBP ≥130 mm Hg and/or DBP ≥85 mm Hg or on treatment for hypertension. 5. High fasting glucose: Plasma glucose level ≥100 mg/dL or on treatment for diabetes.

SUGGESTED READING

1. Bener A, Barışık CC, Acar A, Özdenkaya Y. Assessment of the Gail Model in Estimating the Risk of Breast Cancer: Effect of Cancer Worry and Risk in Healthy Women. Asian Pac J Cancer Prev. 2019;20(6):1765-1771.
2. Cruz-Jentoft AJ, Bahat G, Bauer J, Boirie Y. Sarcopenia: Revised European consensus on definition and diagnosis. Age Ageing. 2019 Jul 1;48(4):601.
3. Heinemann K, Ruebig A, Potthoff P, Schneider HP, Strelow F, Heinemann LA, Do MT. The Menopause Rating Scale (MRS) scale: a methodological review. Health Qual Life Outcomes. 2004;2:45.
4. Lipsy RJ. The National Cholesterol Education Program Adult Treatment Panel III guidelines. J Manag Care Pharm. 2003 Jan-Feb;9(1 Suppl):2-5.
5. Yang M, Hu X, Xie L, et al. Screening Sarcopenia in Community-Dwelling Older Adults: SARC-F vs SARC-F Combined With Calf Circumference (SARC-CalF). J Am Med Dir Assoc. 2018;19(3):277.

2 SECTION

Break the Silence—Not the Bones: A Life Course Management of Osteoporosis

Section Editor: ***Maninder Ahuja***

12 CHAPTER

Pathogenesis of Osteoporosis

Suneeta Mittal

INTRODUCTION

Osteoporosis is compromised bone strength which predisposes to an increased risk of fractures. Bone is continuously being remodeled by osteoblasts (new bone formation) and osteoclasts (bone reabsorption) throughout life. By this process old bone is replaced by new bone. This process continues throughout life, with peak bone mass is reached in third decade of life, with a gradual decline as age advances. When osteoclastic activity is more than osteoblastic activity, osteoporosis occurs. This imbalance is particularly pronounced in postmenopausal women due to estrogen deficiency. Osteoporosis results in decreased bone mineral density (BMD).

CAUSES OF OSTEOPOROSIS

The pathogenesis of osteoporosis is multifactorial, involving a complex interplay of ageing; and genetic, hormonal, metabolic, mechanical, cellular, and immunological factors **(Flowchart 1)**.

1. *Age:* BMD varies throughout life. Bone mass naturally peaks around the third decade and then gradual decline starts. Aging leads to impaired stem cell differentiation into osteoblasts decreasing new bone formation. An increase in marrow adipogenesis can occur with age, which is also associated with reduced bone formation. Not achieving optimal peak bone mass during growth and development also results in osteoporosis as age advances.

Flowchart 1: Overview on pathophysiological mechanisms.

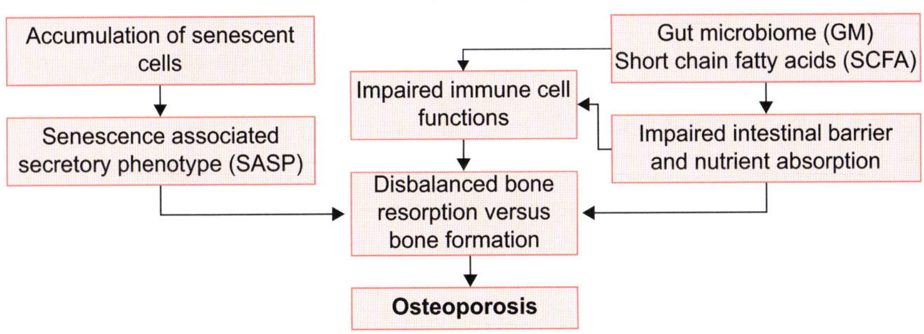

Findings from the mouse model suggest that the adverse effects of old age on the skeleton are independent of estrogens and are due to molecular mechanisms that are distinct from those responsible for the effects of sex steroid deficiency.

Age-related bone loss begins immediately after peak bone mass in men and women, but most bone loss occurs after age of 65 years. In old age is there is increased intracortical porosity which also contributes to bone weakness and fracture risk.

2. *Hormonal factors:* Most important hormone is estrogen, deficiency during postmenopausal period increases osteoclastic activity and accelerates bone resorption resulting in osteoporosis. The onset of cortical bone loss in women is closely linked to estrogen deficiency; however, trabecular bone loss throughout life is mostly age related and estrogen independent. Between menopause and the age of 75 years, women lose approximately 22% of their total body bone mineral, 13.3% is due to aging, and 7.75% is due to estrogen deprivation.

   Other hormones: Parathyroid hormone (PTH), glucocorticoids, thyroid hormones, and androgens also influence bone turnover. Any disease associated with excess of these hormones promotes bone loss.
3. *Genetic and epigenetic factors:* Multiple genes play a significant role affecting bone mass, bone quality, and regulation of bone remodeling pathways. Studies have so far identified approximately 518 genetic loci that influence BMD. A number of these gene loci are involved in Wnt/beta-catenin signaling, the receptor activator of nuclear factor kappa-B ligand (RANKL), osteoprotegerin (OPG) axis, or in mesenchymal cell differentiation.
4. *Cytokines and immune system:* An increase of reactive oxygen species (ROS) in the bone marrow in both aging and estrogen deficiency has been associated with expansion of T and B lymphocytes, nuclear factor kappa-B (NF-κB) activation, and increased production of osteoclastogenic cytokines. Proinflammatory cytokines (e.g., TNF-α, IL-1, and IL-6) and prostaglandin E2, macrophage colony-stimulating factor (M-CSF), and RANKL stimulate osteoclast differentiation and activity, contributing to bone loss. This is called Osteoimmunology. Chronic inflammation, associated with autoimmune diseases, also increases osteoclast-mediated bone resorption.

   The extent to which the effects of estrogens, T and B lymphocytes contribute to the overall antiresorptive effects, and the development of osteoporosis is still unclear.
6. *Oxidative stress:* Oxidative stress is associated with several degenerative disorders associated with aging, including osteoporosis. Both decreased bone formation associated with advancing age, and increased resorption associated with estrogen deficiency is associated with increase in reactive oxygen species (ROS). Increased ROS production in osteoblasts stimulates

apoptosis and decreases bone formation and RANKL—induced osteoclast generation, activation, and survival.

7. *Gut microbiota and metabolic and nutritional factors:* The gut microbiota influences bone health via production of metabolites (e.g., short-chain fatty acids) that modulate immune responses and bone metabolism. Nutritional deficiencies (calcium, vitamin D, and protein) and metabolic disorders (e.g., diabetes) can exacerbate bone loss.
8. *Cellular and molecular pathways:* Osteoclastogenesis is driven by RANKL and modulated by OPG. These are in turn regulated by cytokines and hormones. Increase in RANKL and decrease in OPG a soluble peptide markedly inhibited bone resorption and causes osteoclastic activity, while Osteoblastogenesis is regulated by Wnt/β-catenin signaling. RANKL-induced stimulation of mitochondrial function in osteoclasts also contributes to loss of bone mass. A pathway in the osteoblast-osteoclast interaction scheme is the RANKL—OPG relationship.
9. *Glucocorticoid excess:* Besides ageing and menopause, glucocorticoid excess is a common cause of secondary osteoporosis. Unlike the postmenopausal form of the disease, with use of glucocorticoids the rate of remodeling is low and there is decreased bone formation that decreases bone strength disproportionately with higher risk of fractures. The effects of glucocorticoid excess are direct effects on osteoblasts, osteocytes, and osteoclasts. Changes in the production of local growth factors, including insulin-like growth factors (IGF) and their binding proteins, and Wnt-beta catenin signaling may contribute. There is decrease in angiogenesis resulting from decreased vascular endothelial growth factor (VEGF). Steroid induced osteoporosis is an important cause of low bone mass. Prolonged use of steroids is very common in current era, for many chronic illnesses as well as post-transplant.

   Causes of secondary osteoporosis are listed in **Table 1**.

TABLE 1: Causes for secondary osteoporosis.

Endocrine disorders	Hyperthyroidism, hypogonadism, Cushing's syndrome, type 1 DM, hyperparathyroidism
Nutritional conditions	Malabsorption syndromes and malnutrition, chronic liver disease, gastric operations, Vit D deficiency, calcium deficiency, alcoholism
Drugs	Glucocorticoids, anticonvulsants, gonadotropin-releasing hormone agonists, excessive T4, lithium
Disorders of collagen metabolism	Osteogenesis imperfecta, Homocystinuria, Ehlers-Danlos syndrome, Marfan syndrome
Other	Rheumatoid arthritis, COPD, renal tubular acidosis, hypercalciuria, smoking, organ transplantation, immobilization, mastocytosis

CONCLUSION

Understanding the pathogenesis has important clinical implications for planning therapeutic strategies, including antiresorptive agents (bisphosphonates and denosumab), anabolic agents (teriparatide, abaloparatide, and romosozumab), and potential future therapies targeting mechanosensitive ion channels or osteoimmune pathways. The technical innovations in genetics and proteomics and improved imaging will in future make it possible to have new classes of drugs with specific targets for treating osteoporosis.

KEY POINTS

- Osteoporosis is defined as a skeletal disorder characterized by a compromised bone strength predisposing a person to an increased risk of fracture.
- The epidemiology of osteoporosis is well established, and risk factors have been defined.
- A lifelong, balanced process of old bone removal and new bone creation maintains strength. When this balance is disturbed and osteoclasts work more or osteoblasts do not build enough, net bone loss occurs.
- Osteoporosis is multifactorial. Key factors contributing to osteoporosis include, aging, genetics, hormonal changes, inadequate calcium or Vitamin D, lack of weight-bearing exercise, and corticosteroid use.
- In osteoporosis, there is reduced bone mineral density (BMD), deteriorated microarchitecture, increased bone fragility, and high fracture risk.
- Bone-intrinsic mechanisms, including mitochondria dysfunction, oxidative stress, declining autophagy, DNA damage, osteoprogenitor and osteocyte senescence, senescence-associated secretory phenotype (SASP), and lipid peroxidation, may be primary culprits.
- Bone remodeling occurs throughout life. At a given time, different sites on the bone surface will be in different stages of the remodeling process.

SUGGESTED READING

1. Almeida M, Han L, Ambrogini E, et al. Oxidative stress stimulates apoptosis and activates NF-kappaB in osteoblastic cells via a PKCbeta/p66shc signaling cascade: counter regulation by estrogens or androgens. Mol Endocrinol. 2010;24:2030.
2. Almeida M, Han L, Martin-Millan M, et al. Skeletal involution by age-associated oxidative stress and its acceleration by loss of sex steroids. J Biol Chem. 2007;282:272-85.
3. Bartell SM, Kim HN, Ambrogini E, et al. FoxO proteins restrain osteoclastogenesis and bone resorption by attenuating H2O2 accumulation. Nat Commun. 2014;5:3773.
4. Ding C, Parameswaran V, Udayan R, Burgess J, Jones G. Circulating levels of inflammatory markers predict change in bone mineral density and resorption in older adults: a longitudinal study. J Clin Endocrinol Metab. 2008;93:1952-8.
5. Ding K, Hua F, Ding W. Gut microbiome and osteoporosis. Aging Dis. 2020;11:438-47.

6. Manolagas SC. From estrogen-centric to aging and oxidative stress: a revised perspective of the pathogenesis of osteoporosis. Endocr Rev. 2010;31:266.
7. Morris JA, Kemp JP, Youlten SE, et al. An atlas of genetic influences on osteoporosis in humans and mice. Nat Genet. 2019;51:258.
8. Recker R, Lappe J, Davies K, Heaney R. Characterization of perimenopausal bone loss: a prospective study. J Bone Miner Res. 2000;15:1965.
9. Thacker H. Glucocorticoid-induced Osteoporosis. Cleveland Clinic J Med. 2010;77:843-4.
10. Trajanoska K, Morris JA, Oei L, et al. Assessment of the genetic and clinical determinants of fracture risk: genome wide association and mendelian randomisation study. BMJ. 2018;362:k3225.
11. Ucer S, Iyer S, Kim HN, et al. The Effects of Aging and Sex Steroid Deficiency on the Murine Skeleton Are Independent and Mechanistically Distinct. J Bone Miner Res. 2017;32:560.
12. Van Staa TP, Laan RF, Barton IP, et al. *B*one density threshold and other predictors of vertebral fracture in patients receiving oral glucocorticoid therapy. Arthritis Rheum. 2003;48:3224.
13. Weinstein RS, Nicholas RW, Manolagas SC. Apoptosis of osteocytes in glucocorticoid-induced osteonecrosis of the hip. J Clin Endocrinol Metab. 2000;85:2907.
14. Xiong J, Onal M, Jilka RL, et al. Matrix-embedded cells control osteoclast formation. Nat Med. 2011;17:1235.
15. Zebaze RM, Ghasem-Zadeh A, Bohte A, et al. Intracortical remodelling and porosity in the distal radius and post-mortem femurs of women: a cross-sectional study. Lancet. 2010;375:1729.

13 CHAPTER

Risk Factors for Weak Bones, Magnitude of the Problem

Archana Dwivedi, Saraswathi Kondapalli

Weak bones, including osteopenia and osteoporosis, represent major global public health issues with increasing incidence, rising medical costs, and significant impairment in quality of life. Bone fragility results from the interaction of genetic, nutritional, mechanical, hormonal, and lifestyle factors. Understanding the magnitude of the problem and associated challenges is essential for prevention, early diagnosis, and effective management.

MAGNITUDE OF THE PROBLEM (GLOBAL AND INDIAN PERSPECTIVE)

Worldwide, more than 200 million people are affected by osteoporosis, and a fragility fracture occurs every 3 seconds. Approximately 1 in 3 women and 1 in 5 men above the age of 50 will sustain an osteoporotic fracture in their lifetime. Hip fractures alone account for over 1.6 million cases annually, projected to rise to 6 million by 2050 due to population aging.

Asia is expected to contribute to >50% of all hip fractures by 2050, with India and China being the largest contributors. In India, osteoporosis onset occurs 10–15 years earlier than in Western countries.

National surveys show:

- 70–90% of Indians have vitamin D deficiency, even in sunny regions.
- Average calcium intake is <400 mg/day, far below the recommended requirement.
- High prevalence of early menopause, multiple pregnancies, sedentary lifestyles, and low protein diets further accelerate bone loss.

Fragility fractures in India commonly occur between 55–65 years, compared to 70+ years in Western populations, leading to prolonged disability, loss of productivity, and increased mortality. Hip fracture mortality rates in the first year may reach 20–30%, especially without access to rehabilitation.

RISK FACTORS FOR WEAK BONES

Bone strength depends on peak bone mass achieved by early adulthood and subsequent rate of bone loss. Risk factors can be broadly classified into nonmodifiable, modifiable, and secondary medical causes **(Tables 1 and 2)**.

TABLE 1: Major risk factors for weak bones.

Category	*Risk factors*
Nonmodifiable	Age >50 years, female sex, family history, and thin body frame
Nutritional	Low calcium/vitamin D, low protein, and high phosphorus intake
Lifestyle	Sedentary behavior, smoking, alcohol, and low sun exposure
Hormonal	Early menopause, hypogonadism, and oophorectomy
Medical	RA, CKD, diabetes, liver disease, and malabsorption
Medications	Steroids, PPIs, antiepileptics, and SSRIs

TABLE 2: Early-life versus adult-life risk factors for weak bones.

Stage of life	*Key risk factors*	*Impact*
Childhood	Low calcium diet, limited sunlight, and no sports	Low peak bone mass
Adolescence	Rapid growth without adequate nutrition	Weak skeletal framework
Reproductive age	Multiple pregnancies and anemia	Accelerated nutrient loss
Postmenopause	Estrogen decline and sedentary lifestyle	Rapid bone resorption
Elderly	Sarcopenia, frailty, and poor balance	High fracture risk

Nonmodifiable Risk Factors

- *Age:* Bone mass declines progressively after 40 years, accelerating after menopause due to estrogen deficiency.
- *Sex:* Women are at greater risk because of lower baseline bone mass and abrupt menopause-related bone loss.
- *Genetics:* Family history of fractures or osteoporosis strongly predicts risk.
- *Ethnicity:* Asian and Caucasian populations have higher risk compared to African heritage.
- *Body structure:* Small, thin-framed individuals have lower peak bone mass.

Modifiable Lifestyle Risk Factors

Dietary Factors

Low calcium and vitamin D intake are the most significant contributors. Diets high in refined carbohydrates, low protein, cola drinks (high phosphorus), and poor fruit/vegetable intake impair bone remodeling.

Physical Inactivity

Mechanical loading is essential for bone formation. Sedentary lifestyles, prolonged screen time, and lack of weight-bearing exercise reduce bone stimulation and increase fall risk.

Obesity and Sarcopenia

Although obesity was traditionally considered protective, recent evidence shows that sarcopenic obesity leads to poor balance, impaired bone quality, and greater fracture risk.

Smoking and Alcohol

Nicotine suppresses osteoblasts, while excessive alcohol (>3 drinks/day) induces calcium loss and hormonal imbalance.

Hormonal and Reproductive Factors

- Early menopause (<45 years)
- Surgical menopause
- Long-term lactation without supplementation
- Hypogonadism in men
- Thyroid disorders (especially hyperthyroidism).

Women with multiple closely spaced pregnancies, PCOS with chronic anovulation, or those on long-term steroid contraceptives may also have reduced BMD if nutritional support is inadequate.

Secondary Medical Causes

- Rheumatoid arthritis
- Chronic kidney disease
- Type 1 and 2 diabetes
- Gastrointestinal malabsorption (celiac disease and IBD)
- Chronic liver disease
- Long-term use of steroids, antiepileptics, PPIs, SSRIs, and heparin.

Pathophysiology of Weak Bones

Bone remodeling is a continuous process involving osteoclast-mediated bone resorption and osteoblast-mediated bone formation. With age and exposure to risk factors:

- Resorption exceeds formation → net bone loss
- Trabecular thinning → loss of connectivity
- Cortical porosity increases → decreased mechanical strength
- Altered bone microarchitecture → higher fracture susceptibility

Estrogen deficiency accelerates osteoclast activity, reducing calcium absorption and increasing inflammatory cytokines. Vitamin D deficiency impairs mineralization and causes compensatory secondary hyperparathyroidism.

MAGNITUDE OF THE PROBLEM: ECONOMIC AND SOCIAL BURDEN

Osteoporotic fractures are associated with:

- Prolonged hospitalization
- High surgical costs
- Long-term rehabilitation needs
- Loss of independence
- Increased dependency on caregivers
- Higher risk of institutionalization
- Significant psychological impact (fear of falling and depression).

Global osteoporosis-related healthcare costs exceed USD 37 billion annually. In India, where insurance coverage is limited, families often bear the economic burden.

Peak Bone Mass and Early-life Determinants

Peak bone mass is achieved between 20 and 30 years of age, and nearly 60–80% of one's lifetime bone strength depends on bone accumulation during childhood and adolescence. Factors such as maternal nutrition, birth weight, breastfeeding practices, sunlight exposure, childhood physical activity, and dietary protein intake profoundly influence adult bone health.

Children and adolescents consuming low-dairy diets, high-junk food, and minimal outdoor activity enter adulthood with suboptimal bone reserves. This reduced peak bone mass accelerates the onset of osteopenia, especially in countries like India where:

- Vitamin D deficiency is extremely high even among children
- Early puberty causes early epiphyseal closure
- Academic pressure reduces outdoor activity
- Urban pollution limits UVB availability.

Thus, bone fragility in adulthood often begins silently during early growth years.

Understanding Bone Quality versus Bone Density

Most screening methods assess bone mineral density (BMD), but bone strength also depends on:

- Collagen cross-linking
- Trabecular connectivity
- Cortical thickness

- Microcracks and turnover rate
- Bone material properties (BMP)

Normal BMD does not rule out fracture risk in:
- Type 2 diabetes
- Long-term steroid use
- Chronic inflammatory diseases
- Postmenopausal women with rapid bone turnover.

Therefore, bone quality assessment using TBS (Trabecular Bone Score), HR-pQCT, or bone turnover markers is increasingly recognized as essential in advanced clinical settings.

Sex-specific Considerations

Women

Women experience rapid bone loss due to estrogen decline. Additional contributors include:
- Multiple pregnancies with inadequate calcium
- High prevalence of anemia and low protein diets
- Early surgical menopause due to hysterectomy + oophorectomy
- Breastfeeding without supplementation.

Men

Men are often underdiagnosed, because osteoporosis is perceived as a "women's disease." However, mortality after hip fractures is significantly higher in men. Hypogonadism, alcohol dependence, smoking, and chronic illnesses contribute heavily to bone loss in males.

Challenges in Addressing Weak Bones (Table 3)

- *Lack of awareness:* Osteoporosis is a "silent disease." Most patients remain asymptomatic until fractures occur. Awareness about vitamin D, calcium, and weight-bearing exercise is limited.
- *Underdiagnosis:* DXA scan availability is limited in smaller towns. Vertebral fractures are often missed, because they may be painless.

TABLE 3: Key challenges in prevention and management.

Challenge	*Impact*
Poor awareness	Late diagnosis, fractures occur before detection
Limited DXA access	Underestimation of disease burden
Low treatment adherence	Higher refracture risk
Nutritional deficits	Reduced peak bone mass
Lack of fall-prevention programs	Increased hip fractures

- *Treatment gaps:* Even after a fragility fracture, fewer than 20% of patients receive osteoporosis treatment. Concerns about medication side effects (especially bisphosphonates) lead to poor adherence.
- *Nutritional deficiencies:* Cultural diets low in dairy, vegetarianism, and fast-food consumption contribute to widespread calcium and protein deficiency.
- *Hormonal and metabolic disorders:* Poor screening for thyroid disorders, CKD, celiac disease, and early menopause increases missed diagnoses.
- *Fall risk:* Poor vision, improper footwear, cluttered homes, neuropathy, and sarcopenia lead to preventable falls.
- *Health system-based challenges:*
    - Lack of fracture liaison services (FLS) that ensure structured treatment after the first fracture.
    - Limited geriatric care specialization in many developing countries.
    - Poor integration between orthopedic, gynecology, and endocrine departments.
    - Inconsistent availability of DXA scans in semiurban and rural hospitals.
- *Patient behavior challenges:*
    - Discontinuation of therapy due to lack of symptoms.
    - Misconceptions about "weight gain" from calcium tablets.
    - Preference for unproven herbal products instead of medical management.
    - Fear of injectable treatments.
- *Socioeconomic challenges:*
    - Low affordability of advanced medications like teriparatide or romosozumab.
    - Low insurance coverage for chronic bone diseases.
    - Dietary gaps caused by rising food prices.

CONCLUSION

Weak bones represent a major global health concern with increasing prevalence in aging populations. Both modifiable and nonmodifiable risk factors contribute to reduced bone strength, while socioeconomic barriers and limited awareness hinder early diagnosis. Addressing nutritional deficiencies, improving screening access, implementing fall-prevention strategies, and enhancing treatment adherence are crucial steps. A comprehensive public health approach integrating lifestyle, nutrition, medical therapy, and community awareness is essential to reduce the burden of fractures and associated disability.

SUGGESTED READING

1. Adachi JD et al. Clin Ther. 2003.
2. Binkley N et al. J Clin Densitom. 2008.
3. Compston JE. Clin Endocrinol. 2019.
4. Cooper C et al. Am J Med. 1997.
5. Cummings SR, Melton LJ. Lancet. 2002.
6. Das S et al. Indian J Med Res. 2021.
7. Eastell R et al. Lancet Diabetes Endocrinol. 2016.
8. Ensrud KE et al. Arch Intern Med. 1997.
9. Harinarayan CV. J Clin Endocrinol Metab. 2014.
10. Johnell O, Kanis JA. Osteoporos Int. 2006.
11. Kanis JA et al. Osteoporos Int. 2013.
12. Khadilkar A et al. Osteoporos Int. 2018.
13. Looker AC et al. J Bone Miner Res. 2012.
14. Mithal A et al. Osteoporos Int. 2009.
15. Modi A et al. Osteoporos Int. 2019.
16. Nguyen TV et al. J Bone Miner Res. 1995.
17. Reginster JY, Burlet N. Bone. 2006.
18. Rizzoli R et al. Osteoporos Int. 2014.
19. Sambrook P, Cooper C. Lancet. 2006.
20. World Health Organization. WHO Technical Report. 2003.

14 CHAPTER

Role of Estrogen in Postmenopausal Osteoporosis

Ruchika Garg

EPIDEMIOLOGY OF POSTMENOPAUSAL OSTEOPOROSIS

Osteoporosis affects a substantial proportion of women beyond the age of 50 years worldwide, with postmenopausal estrogen deficiency being a dominant risk factor. Fragility fractures are associated with chronic pain, deformity, loss of independence, and excess mortality, especially after hip and multiple vertebral fractures, making primary and secondary prevention a major public health priority.

Estrogen plays a central role in the pathogenesis, prevention, and treatment of osteoporosis at menopause. Its decline during menopause is the primary driver of accelerated bone loss, leading to increased fracture risk and significant morbidity in postmenopausal women. This chapter synthesizes current evidence on the mechanisms, clinical impact, and therapeutic role of estrogen in menopausal osteoporosis.

PATHOPHYSIOLOGY: ESTROGEN AND BONE REMODELING

Bone is a dynamic tissue maintained by a balance between osteoclast-mediated resorption and osteoblast-driven formation. Estrogen is the dominant sex hormone responsible for preserving bone mass in women. Its deficiency at menopause disrupts this equilibrium, resulting in a high-turnover state characterized by disproportionate loss of trabecular bone, cortical thinning, and deterioration of bone quality.

Estrogen maintains skeletal homeostasis by tightly coupling bone resorption and formation. It suppresses osteoclastogenesis primarily by downregulating receptor activator of nuclear factor κB ligand (RANKL) and upregulating osteoprotegerin (OPG) in osteoblasts, osteocytes, and bone-lining cells. This limits osteoclast recruitment, activity, and survival. After menopause, the sharp fall in estrogen shifts the RANKL/OPG ratio in favor of RANKL, enhancing osteoclast differentiation through RANK on osteoclast precursors and accelerating bone resorption.

Estrogen also exerts direct and indirect effects on bone cells and the bone microenvironment. It enhances osteoclast apoptosis by increasing transforming growth factor-β and Fas ligand signaling from osteoblast-lineage cells, and reduces oxidative stress and inflammatory cytokines that promote bone resorption. Additionally, estrogen supports osteoblast and osteocyte survival, maintains lacunar-canalicular integrity, and limits microdamage accumulation, contributing to bone strength beyond effects on bone mineral density (BMD) alone **(Flowchart 1 and Table 1)**.

Fracture risk assessment tools such as FRAX incorporate age, BMD, prior fracture, and clinical risk factors. However, large trial analyses demonstrate that the relative fracture-risk reduction with menopausal hormone therapy (MHT) is largely independent of baseline FRAX probability or falls history. This implies that appropriately selected postmenopausal women across a

Flowchart 1: Role of estrogen in menopausal osteoporosis.

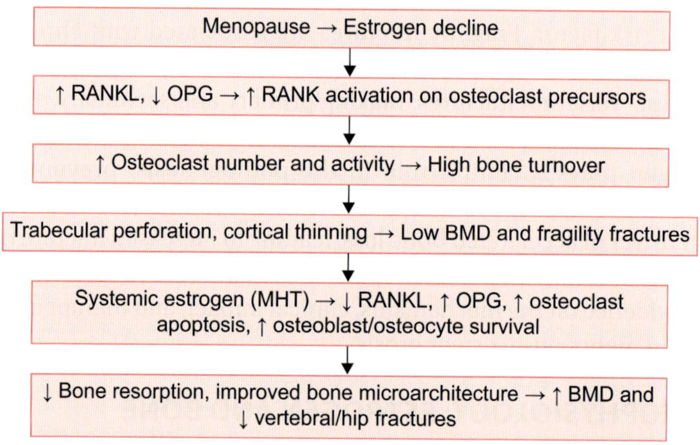

TABLE 1: Estrogen in menopausal osteoporosis.

Aspect	*Key points*
Pathophysiological role	Estrogen deficiency after menopause increases RANKL and decreases OPG, enhancing osteoclastogenesis and bone resorption
Skeletal consequences	Rapid loss of trabecular and cortical bone, microarchitectural deterioration, and increased vertebral and hip fracture risk
Efficacy of MHT	Standard-dose MHT increases BMD and reduces all fractures by ≈28% and hip fractures by ≈34% in postmenopausal women
Ideal candidates	Symptomatic women within 10 years of menopause or <60 years, or women with premature menopause, with increased fracture risk and no major contraindications
Route and regimen	All systemic routes are effective. Progestogen is required if the uterus is present
Position vs. other drugs	Considered first line for early postmenopausal women with symptoms and raised fracture risk; nonestrogen agents preferred for older or very high-risk women

spectrum of baseline risk can derive skeletal benefit from estrogen-containing regimens, although absolute benefit is greater in those at higher baseline risk.

MECHANISMS OF RAPID POSTMENOPAUSAL BONE LOSS

The timeline of postmenopausal bone loss is characterized by distinct phases:

- *Year 0–1:* Trabecular bone loss predominates (cancellous bone has higher turnover).
- *Year 1–5:* Accelerated phase → loss of entire trabeculae → irreversible architecture damage.
- *Year 5+:* Slower cortical thinning + continued endocortical resorption.

Net result: Women lose ~35–50% of trabecular and ~25–30% of cortical bone lifetime.

CLINICAL EVIDENCE: ESTROGEN AND FRACTURE REDUCTION

Randomized trials and large observational studies consistently show that estrogen therapy, alone or combined with a progestogen in women with a uterus, increases BMD and reduces fractures. Data from the Women's Health Initiative (WHI) and other major trials demonstrate that combined conjugated estrogens plus medroxyprogesterone acetate reduce hip fractures by about 34% and all clinical fractures by approximately 24–30% compared with placebo, regardless of baseline BMD.

Menopausal hormone therapy lowers the risk of any fracture by around 28% and hip fracture by about 34%, with similar relative risk reductions across different FRAX-predicted baseline risks and irrespective of falls history. Standard-dose estrogen or estrogen-progestin therapy increases bone mass mainly by decreasing bone turnover, and that the protective effect persists while therapy is continued, with partial attenuation after discontinuation but no rebound excess fracture risk compared with never-users.

INDICATIONS AND PLACE OF ESTROGEN THERAPY

Menopausal hormone therapy is a cost-effective first-line option for prevention and early treatment of postmenopausal osteoporosis in symptomatic women within 10 years of menopause and below about 60 years of age, provided there are no contraindications. Estrogen therapy is also the primary modality for bone protection in women with premature ovarian insufficiency or early menopause and should generally be continued at least until the average age of natural menopause **(Fig. 1)**.

In major clinical practice guidelines for postmenopausal osteoporosis, nonestrogen agents such as bisphosphonates, denosumab, or anabolic therapies are recommended as first-line in older women at very high

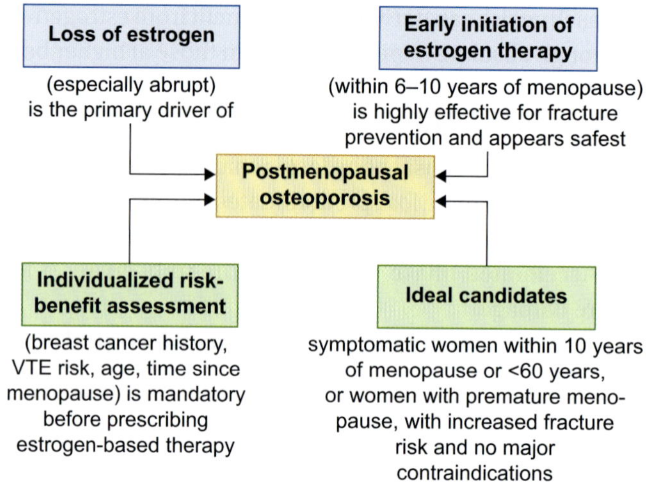

Fig. 1: Place of estrogen therapy.

Flowchart 2: Clinical use of estrogen in osteoporosis at menopause.

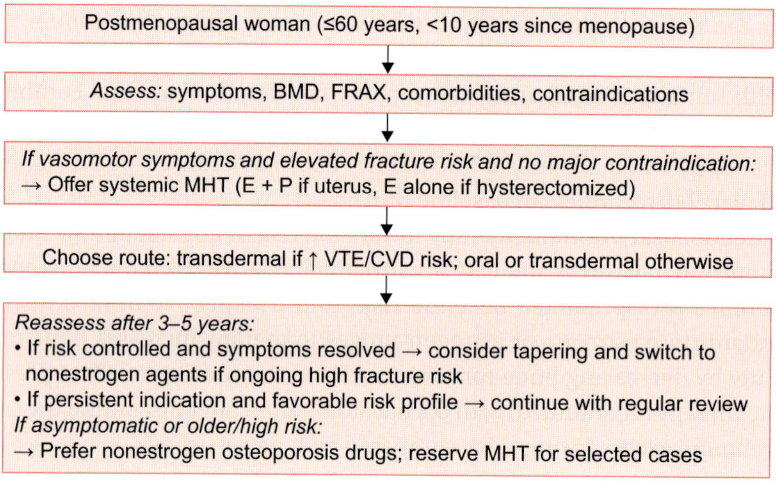

fracture risk, whereas MHT is considered an appropriate option for younger, early postmenopausal women who also have vasomotor or genitourinary symptoms and an elevated fracture risk profile **(Flowchart 2 and Table 2)**.

REGIMENS, ROUTES, AND DURATION

All standard systemic estrogen preparations—oral, transdermal, and other nonoral formulations—are effective for preserving or increasing BMD when used at adequate doses. Transdermal estradiol is often preferred for women at increased risk of venous thromboembolism, stroke, or cardiovascular disease, as it avoids first-pass hepatic metabolism and exerts less effect on coagulation and triglycerides **(Fig. 2)**.

TABLE 2: Estrogen-based and estrogen-mimicking therapies.

Agent	*Class*	*Route*	*Effect on bone*	*Approved indications*
Conjugated equine estrogens (CEE)	Natural estrogen mix	Oral	Strong antifracture efficacy	Menopausal symptoms, osteoporosis prevention
17β-estradiol	Bioidentical	Trans-dermal, vaginal	Same efficacy, lower VTE risk	Same + local vaginal atrophy
Bazedoxifene + CEE	Tissue-Selective Estrogen Complex (TSEC)	Oral	+BMD, no endometrial hyperplasia	Menopausal symptoms, osteoporosis prevention
Raloxifene	SERM (second generation)	Oral	+2–3% BMD, 30–40% vertebral fx ↓	Postmenopausal osteoporosis, breast Ca risk ↓
Tibolone	STEAR (metabolites have E, P, A activity)	Oral	+BMD, fewer hot flushes	Europe/Asia (not FDA-approved)

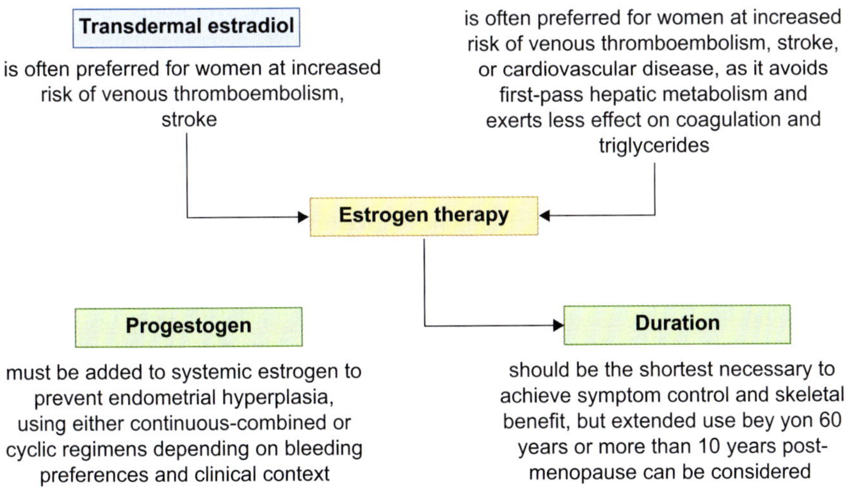

Fig. 2: How to prescribe estrogen therapy.

In women with an intact uterus, progestogen must be added to systemic estrogen to prevent endometrial hyperplasia therapies.

CONCLUSION

Estrogen plays a central role in the pathogenesis, prevention, and treatment of osteoporosis at menopause, and appropriately selected menopausal hormone therapy (MHT) remains one of the most effective options for early postmenopausal women at increased fracture risk. Individualized assessment, careful selection, and periodic review are essential to maximize benefits and minimize risks.

SUGGESTED READING

1. ACOG Committee Opinion No. 698. Hormone therapy in primary ovarian insufficiency. Obstet Gynecol. 2017;129(5):e134–41.
2. Cauley JA, Robbins J, Chen Z, et al. Effects of estrogen plus progestin on risk of fracture and bone mineral density: The Women's Health Initiative randomized trial. JAMA. 2003;290(13):1729-38.
3. Eastell R, Rosen CJ, Black DM, et al. Pharmacological management of osteoporosis in postmenopausal women: An Endocrine Society guideline. J Clin Endocrinol Metab. 2019;104(5):1595-622.
4. Frontiers in Reproductive Health. Impact of menopause hormone therapy, exercise, and their combination on bone mineral density in menopausal osteoporosis. Front Reprod Health. 2025;2:1542746.
5. Harvey NC, McCloskey EV, Kanis JA, et al. New insights into hormone replacement therapy for preventing fractures. Osteoporos Int. 2022;33(5):923-31.
6. Lorentzon M, Johansson H, Harvey NC, et al. Menopausal hormone therapy reduces fracture risk regardless of FRAX probability and falls history. Osteoporos Int. 2022;33(9):1919-29.
7. Medscape. Menopausal hormone therapy: Overview, symptoms, and effects. [online] Available from https://emedicine.medscape.com/article/276104-overview?form=fpf [Last accessed January, 2026].
8. Nambiar V, et al. Postmenopausal osteoporosis: Menopause hormone therapy and other management options. J Midlife Health. 2023;14(4):233-42.
9. Pace DT, et al. Estrogen hormone therapy and postmenopausal osteoporosis. Climacteric. 2023;26(6):1-10.
10. Royal Osteoporosis Society. Hormone replacement therapy (HRT): Osteoporosis. [online] Available from https://theros.org.uk/information-and-support/osteoporosis/treatment/hormone-replacement-therapy/ [Last accessed January, 2026].
11. Streicher C, Heyny A, Andrukhova O, et al. Estrogen regulates bone turnover by targeting RANKL expression in bone lining cells. JCI Insight. 2017;2(6):e91142.
12. Tera TM, do Prado RF, DE Marco AC, et al. RANKL/OPG interaction in bone loss after estrogen deficiency. Braz Oral Res. 2014;28(1):1-9.
13. Tobeiha M, Moghadasian MH, Amin N, et al. RANKL/RANK/OPG pathway: A mechanism involved in exercise-induced bone remodeling. Front Physiol. 2020;11:1-16.
14. Vinogradova Y, Coupland C, Hippisley-Cox J. Discontinuation of menopausal hormone therapy and risk of fracture: A population-based study. Lancet Healthy Longev. 2025;6(7):e500-12.
15. Watts NB, Cauley JA, Jackson RD, et al. No increase in fractures after stopping hormone therapy: Findings from the Women's Health Initiative. J Clin Endocrinol Metab. 2017;102(1):302-10.

15 CHAPTER

Crosstalk Between Osteoporosis and Sarcopenia

Binal Shah

INTRODUCTION

Osteoporosis and sarcopenia are two major musculoskeletal disorders prevalent in older adults. While traditionally viewed as distinct conditions—one affecting bone and the other muscle—current evidence emphasizes that they are biologically interconnected and often co-exist as "osteosarcopenia." This overlap results in greater functional impairment, frailty, falls, fractures, disability, and mortality than either condition alone.

The biological crosstalk between bone and muscle occurs through mechanical, biochemical, endocrine, and molecular pathways. Understanding these interactions is crucial for developing integrated preventive and therapeutic strategies.

DEFINITIONS

Osteoporosis

A systemic skeletal disorder characterized by:

- Low bone mass
- Microarchitectural deterioration of bone tissue
- Increased bone fragility and fracture risk

Diagnosis (WHO criteria): T-score ≤ -2.5 SD at the femoral neck or lumbar spine.

Sarcopenia

A progressive and generalized skeletal muscle disorder involving:

- Loss of muscle mass
- Reduced muscle strength
- Impaired physical performance

Diagnosis (EWGSOP$_2$ criteria):

- *Probable sarcopenia:* Low muscle strength
- *Confirmed sarcopenia:* Low strength + low muscle mass
- *Severe sarcopenia:* Above + poor physical performance

Osteosarcopenia

The coexistence of osteoporosis and sarcopenia, accompanied by a synergistic decline in musculoskeletal health resulting in increased vulnerability to falls and fractures.

EPIDEMIOLOGY

- Both conditions increase with aging and are more common in women.
- Sarcopenia affects ~10–20% of adults ≥65 years.
- Osteoporosis affects >200 million individuals globally.
- Osteosarcopenia prevalence ranges from 5 to 37% in community-dwelling older adults and up to 50% in institutionalized populations.
- Coexistence greatly amplifies fracture risk (2–4× compared with osteoporosis alone).

SHARED RISK FACTORS

Both disorders share several modifiable and nonmodifiable risk factors:

Nonmodifiable factors:

- Aging
- Female sex
- Genetics
- Hormonal changes (menopause, andropause)

Modifiable factors:

- Physical inactivity
- Poor nutrition (low protein, calcium, and vitamin D)
- Chronic diseases (diabetes, rheumatoid arthritis, and COPD)
- Medications (glucocorticoids and aromatase inhibitors)
- Chronic inflammation

MECHANISMS OF CROSSTALK BETWEEN BONE AND MUSCLE

Mechanical Crosstalk

Muscle loading is a primary driver of bone formation. Reduced muscle mass or strength leads to:

- Decreased mechanical strain
- Reduced bone formation
- Lower bone mineral density (BMD)

Endocrine and Biochemical Crosstalk

Muscle-derived myokines that affect bone:

- *Myostatin:* Inhibits muscle growth; increases bone resorption

- *Irisin:* Promotes osteoblast differentiation
- *IL-6 (acute):* Supports bone remodeling
- *IGF-1:* Enhances bone anabolic activity

Bone-derived osteokines that influence muscle:

- *Osteocalcin (undercarboxylated):* Stimulates muscle glucose uptake and performance
- *Sclerostin:* Inhibits Wnt signaling → decreased muscle and bone formation
- *FGF23:* Impacts muscle metabolism indirectly via phosphate regulation

Chronic Low-grade Inflammation

Inflammaging (elevated IL-6, TNF-α, and CRP):

- Promotes muscle protein breakdown
- Stimulates osteoclastogenesis → bone loss

Hormonal Pathways

- Decline in estrogen/testosterone reduces both bone and muscle mass.
- Growth hormone and IGF-1 deficiency impair protein synthesis and bone formation.
- Vitamin D deficiency affects muscle contraction and bone mineralization.

Mitochondrial Dysfunction

Shared mitochondrial and metabolic alterations in aging muscle and bone drive:

- Reduced energy production
- Increased reactive oxygen species (ROS)
- Accelerated tissue atrophy

Neuromuscular Dysfunction

Loss of motor neurons contributes to muscle atrophy, reduced mechanical loading, and secondary bone loss.

CLINICAL IMPACT OF THE OSTEOPOROSIS–SARCOPENIA INTERACTION

Increased Fracture Risk

The combination of weak muscles and fragile bones significantly elevates fracture risk:

- Higher fall incidence
- Impaired postural stability
- Reduced protective reflexes

Functional Decline

- Difficulty in ADLs (activities of daily living)
- Reduced gait speed
- Fatigue and reduced endurance

Increased Morbidity and Mortality

Hip fractures in osteosarcopenic individuals have worse outcomes and higher 1-year mortality.

Higher Health-care Utilization

- Longer hospitalizations
- Greater need for institutional care or rehabilitation

DIAGNOSIS AND ASSESSMENT

Osteoporosis

- *DXA scan:* BMD at lumbar spine, femoral neck
- *FRAX score:* Estimated fracture risk
- Vertebral fracture assessment

Sarcopenia

- *Muscle strength:* Handgrip strength and chair stand test
- *Muscle mass:* DXA, bioimpedance analysis (BIA), and CT/MRI
- *Physical performance:* Gait speed, TUG test, and SPPB

Osteosarcopenia

Identified when both low BMD and low muscle mass/strength/performance coexist.

TREATMENT STRATEGIES

Exercise (Cornerstone Therapy)

For both osteoporosis and sarcopenia:

- Progressive resistance training (2–3×/week)
- Weight-bearing aerobic activities
- Balance and functional training
- High-intensity interval training (where appropriate)

Benefits:

- Increases muscle mass and strength
- Improves BMD
- Reduces falls
- Enhances physical function

Nutritional Interventions

Protein:

- Recommend 1.0–1.2 g/kg/day (up to 1.5 g/kg/day in frail elderly)
- Leucine-rich sources to stimulate muscle protein synthesis

Vitamin D:

- Target 25(OH)D >30 ng/mL
- Supplementation 800–1,000 IU/day if deficient

Calcium: 1,000–1,200 mg/day (diet + supplements)

Creatine: Improves muscle strength and may indirectly support bone health

Omega-3 fatty acids: Reduces inflammation and enhances anabolic response

Pharmacological Therapy

Drugs for osteoporosis:

- Antiresorptives: Bisphosphonates and denosumab
- Anabolics: Teriparatide, abaloparatide, and romosozumab. Some anabolic agents also improve muscle function.

Emerging agents targeting both tissues:

- Myostatin inhibitors
- Selective androgen receptor modulators (SARMs)
- Sclerostin inhibitors

TABLE 1: Key differences and overlap between osteoporosis and sarcopenia.

Feature	*Osteoporosis*	*Sarcopenia*	*Osteosarcopenia (overlap)*
Primary tissue affected	Bone	Muscle	Both
Core pathology	Low BMD, microarchitectural deterioration	Loss of muscle mass, strength	Combined bone fragility + muscle weakness
Key drivers	Hormonal decline, inactivity	Anabolic resistance, poor nutrition	Shared endocrine, metabolic,
Main consequences	Fragility fractures	Falls, disability	High fracture risk, severe disability
Main diagnostic tool	DXA (BMD)	Grip strength, gait speed, muscle mass (DXA/BIA)	Combined criteria
Treatment focus	Anti-resorptives, anabolics	Resistance training, protein	

Fall Prevention

- Home safety evaluation
- Vision correction
- Assistive devices
- Medication review

TABLE 2: Tools for musculoskeletal evaluation.

Component	*Test*	*Interpretation*
Bone mass	DXA (T-score)	≤ −2.5: Osteoporosis
Muscle mass	DXA appendicular lean mass, CT, MRI	Low ALM/height^2
Muscle strength	Handgrip dynamometery	<27 kg (men), <16 kg (women)
Performance	Gait speed, chair stand test	<0.8 m/s = poor performance

CONCLUSION

Understanding the crosstalk between osteoporosis and sarcopenia has transformed the perception of musculoskeletal aging. Instead of isolated conditions, they represent interlinked pathologies driven by shared biological mechanisms. Recognizing and treating osteosarcopenia as a unified clinical entity enables more effective prevention of falls, fractures, disability, and loss of independence. Comprehensive strategies that combine exercise, nutrition, pharmacotherapy, and fall prevention represent the best approach to preserving musculoskeletal health across the lifespan.

KEY POINTS

- Osteoporosis and sarcopenia frequently coexist and share many risk factors.
- They communicate through mechanical loading, hormonal pathways, myokines, and osteokines.
- Osteosarcopenia leads to significantly higher rates of falls, fractures, disability, and mortality.
- Diagnosis requires combined assessment of bone mass and muscle strength/mass.
- Resistance training and adequate protein/vitamin D intake form the cornerstone of management.
- Emerging drugs targeting both bone and muscle (e.g., myostatin inhibitors and sclerostin inhibitors) show promise.
- An interdisciplinary approach is required for effective prevention and treatment.

KEY MESSAGES

1. Bone and muscle are not independent tissues; they form an integrated functional unit whose decline with age is interdependent.
2. Osteosarcopenia is a high-risk condition associated with markedly increased fractures and mortality.

3. Chronic inflammation, hormonal decline, mechanical unloading, and endocrine signaling mediate the bone–muscle crosstalk.
4. Early diagnosis is critical, as both conditions often remain silent until a fall or fracture occurs.
5. Exercise—particularly resistance training—is the most effective nonpharmacological therapy for both conditions.
6. Nutritional optimization (protein, calcium, vitamin D) is essential for maintaining muscle and bone health.
7. Future therapies will increasingly target the shared pathways of bone and muscle degeneration.
8. Integrated interventions outperform single-focus treatments, highlighting the need for combined management strategies.

SUGGESTED READING

1. Binkley N, Krueger D, Buehring B. What's in a name revisited: should osteoporosis and sarcopenia be considered components of "dysmobility syndrome"? Osteoporos Int. 2013;24(12):2955-9.
2. Brotto M, Johnson ML. Endocrine crosstalk between muscle and bone. Curr Osteoporos Rep. 2014;12(2):135-41.
3. Cruz-Jentoft AJ, Bahat G, Bauer J, et al. Sarcopenia: revised European consensus on definition and diagnosis. Age Ageing. 2019;48(1):16-31.
4. Eastell R, Rosen CJ, Black DM, et al. Pharmacological management of osteoporosis in postmenopausal women. Lancet. 2019;393(10169):791-804.
5. Hirschfeld HP, Kinsella R, Duque G. Osteosarcopenia: where bone, muscle, and fat collide. Osteoporos Int. 2017;28:2781-90.
6. Kanis JA, Cooper C, Rizzoli R, et al. European guidance for the diagnosis and management of osteoporosis. Osteoporos Int. 2019;30:3-44.
7. Kirk B, Zanker J, Duque G. Osteosarcopenia: epidemiology, diagnosis, and treatment—facts and numbers. J Cachexia Sarcopenia Muscle. 2020;11(3):609-18.
8. Landi F, Liperoti R, Russo A, et al. Sarcopenia as a risk factor for falls in elderly individuals: results from the ilSIRENTE study. Clin Nutr. 2012;31(5):652-8.
9. Rolph DN, Deban JF, Visser M. The role of nutrition in sarcopenia and frailty. Curr Opin Clin Nutr Metab Care. 2021;24(1):20-6.
10. Tagliaferri C, Wittrant Y, Davicco MJ, et al. Muscle and bone, two interconnected tissues. Ageing Res Rev. 2015;21:55-70.

16 CHAPTER

Attainment of Adolescent PBM and Prevention of Osteoporosis

Uma Vaidyanathan

ADOLESCENT PREVENTION OF OSTEOPOROSIS

INTRODUCTION

Bone is a dynamic living tissue, continually renewed throughout life. This turnover is most active in childhood—nearly 20% of the skeleton remodels each year in growing children compared with just 3–5% in adults. Osteoporosis, defined in adults as a BMD T-score ≤–2.5 SD, represents a reduction in bone mass and deterioration in bone microarchitecture, ultimately increasing fracture susceptibility.

Although typically diagnosed later in life, the foundation for future bone strength is largely set during adolescence.

Adolescence (10–19 years) is a phase marked by rapid skeletal growth, hormonal changes, and evolving lifestyle patterns. Nearly all modifiable factors that influence lifelong bone health—diet, sunlight exposure, activity level, body weight, and menstrual health—take shape during these years.

WHY ADOLESCENCE MATTERS FOR BONE HEALTH

Peak Bone Mass Accrual

- Approximately 40–60% of adult bone mass is accumulated during adolescence.
- Almost one-quarter of peak bone mass (PBM) is achieved during the short pubertal growth spurt.
- Attaining optimal PBM lowers lifetime fracture risk by nearly 50%.
- Girls complete PBM earlier (16–18 years), while boys continue into early adulthood.

So, those who reach a lower peak bone mass in early twenties are going to end up with a much lower bone mass in their old age beyond the 50s.

Hormonal Influences

- Estrogen supports epiphyseal maturation, boosts calcium absorption, and reduces bone resorption.

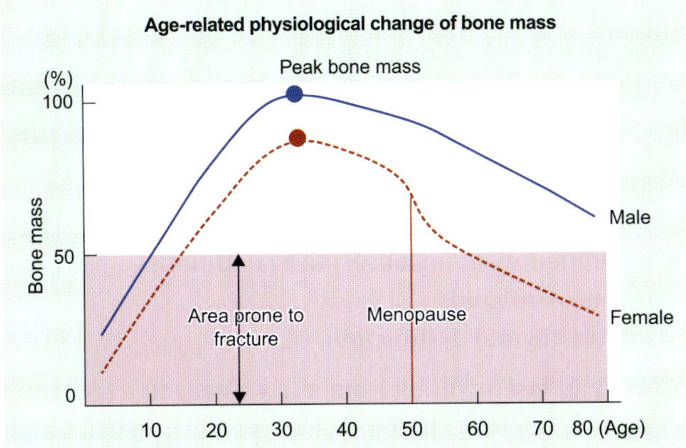

Fig. 1: There is a tremendous amount of increase in bone mass from birth to the young adult age. The bone mineral deposition accelerates manyfold during the puberty for 3 to 4 years and the peak bone mass is attained usually by the early 20s. After the peak bone mass is achieved, there is a gradual reduction in bone mass during the adult age by around 0.5–1% per year. This bone loss accelerates in older age and is much faster in women after menopause, reaching a loss of 2–5% bone mass per year in the initial 5–7 years after menopause due to lack of estrogen.

- Testosterone improves muscle bulk, enhancing mechanical loading and stimulating bone formation.
- GH and IGF-1 remain high during puberty, accelerating bone turnover.

Lifestyle Evolution

- Adolescents often shift toward discretionary diets.
- Increased screen time reduces outdoor activity and sunlight exposure.
- Frequent meal skipping, poor dairy intake, and rising consumption of processed foods are common patterns.

RISK FACTORS FOR POOR BONE ACCRUAL IN ADOLESCENCE

Nutritional

- Low calcium intake (<1,000 mg/day)
- Vitamin D deficiency—reported in >70% of Indian adolescents
- Insufficient protein (<1 g/kg/day)
- High soft-drink consumption; phosphoric acid may negatively affect BMD
- Excess caffeine (>2 cups/day)

Lifestyle

- Sedentary routine (screen time >3–4 hours/day)
- Inadequate sports participation; overtraining and RED-S in athletes

- Indoor lifestyle with limited sunlight
- Early initiation of smoking or alcohol.

Medical

- Delayed puberty, hypogonadism
- Eating disorders—anorexia or bulimia
- Chronic inflammatory or malabsorptive conditions
- Long-term glucocorticoids
- Type 1 diabetes, thyroid dysfunction.

Peak growth can last anything from a few weeks to a few months. Good nutrition (especially calcium, vitamin D, and protein), regular weight-bearing exercise, and avoidance of smoking or extreme dieting during this period directly improve peak bone mass, which protects against osteoporosis and fractures in adulthood.

Anthropometric

- BMI <18.5 kg/m^2
- Restrictive diets/rapid weight loss
- Obesity—associated with vitamin D deficiency and poor mobility.

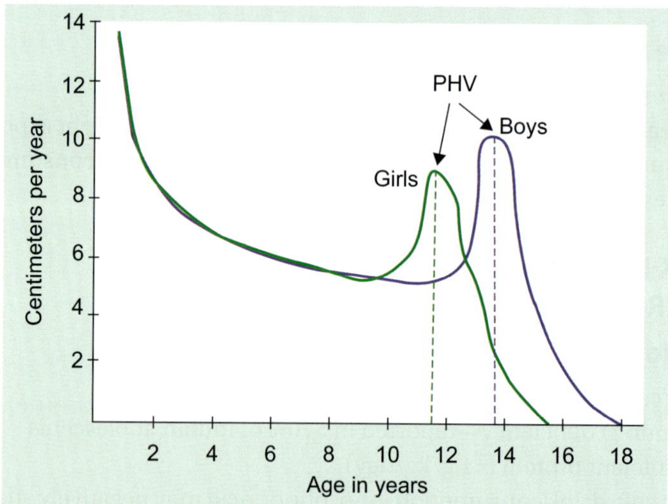

Fig. 2: Peak height velocity (PHV) is a period in childhood where maximum rate of growth occurs. It is otherwise known as the Growth Spurt. It indicates hormonal, physiological, and anatomical changes in the body bringing a child into adolescence. Although children may have a few smaller secondary growth spurts, PHV usually occurs as a single event. This usually takes place few years earlier in girls (10–12 years old) than boys (12–14 years old).

RED FLAGS REQUIRING CLINICAL EVALUATION

- Multiple fractures → evaluate for metabolic bone disease
- Delayed puberty → possible hormonal insufficiency
- Menstrual irregularities or >3 months of amenorrhea → low estrogen compromising bone health
- BMI <18.5 kg/m^2 or marked weight loss → risk of disordered eating
- Chronic illness → impaired bone formation
- Long-term steroids → secondary osteoporosis.

EVIDENCE-BASED PREVENTION STRATEGIES

Nutrition

Calcium:

- *Requirement:* 1,000–1,300 mg/day
- *Sources:* Milk, curd, paneer, ragi, sesame, amaranth, and fortified foods
- Aim for 2–3 dairy servings daily.

Vitamin D:

- *Requirement:* 600–1,000 IU/day
- *Sun exposure:* 15–20 minutes mid-morning to arms and face
- *Foods:* Fortified milk, mushrooms, fish, and egg yolk
- Routine supplementation is often necessary in India.

Protein:

- *Needs:* 1.0–1.2 g/kg/day
- Mixed animal–plant protein improves bone matrix deposition.

Other Micronutrients

Magnesium, phosphorus, vitamin K, and zinc support mineralization and collagen formation.

Dietary Advice

- Minimize carbonated drinks and high-salt snacks.
- Encourage nuts, fruits, and yoghurt as alternatives.
- Promote traditional Indian calcium-rich meals.

Physical Activity

Weight-bearing activity:

- Crucial for bone modelling and strength.
- Adolescents require 60 min/day of activity including:
  - *Impact exercises:* Jumping, skipping, and running
  - *Sports:* Basketball, football, martial arts, and gymnastics
- Resistance training 2–3 times/week improves BMD.

Reducing sedentary time:

- Limit screen time to <2 hours/day.
- Promote outdoor play and organized sports.

Lifestyle Behaviors

Avoid smoking and alcohol: Both impair bone turnover, hormonal stability, and calcium balance.

Sleep: 8–10 hours supports the GH–IGF pathway essential for bone growth.

Healthy weight:

- Maintain normal BMI.
- Early recognition of disordered eating is essential.

Screening and Early Detection

DEXA is not recommended routinely. Use selective screening for:

- Two long-bone fractures
- Steroid use
- Amenorrhea >6 months
- Chronic systemic disease
- Eating disorders

Tools include:

- Dietary recall, activity questionnaires
- Growth charts, Tanner staging
- Menstrual history

Interventions for low BMD:

- Calcium + Vitamin D supplementation
- Planned exercise program
- Treat underlying disease
- Lifestyle counseling

School, Family, and Community Approaches

School-based:

- Nutrition modules
- Daily sports periods
- Healthy canteen guidelines
- Screening for menstrual irregularities

Family-based:

- Family meals high in calcium
- Outdoor weekend activities
- Device-free time to reduce screen exposure

Public health:

- Vitamin D fortification
- Safe neighborhood parks
- Awareness programs

Special Situations

Girls:

- Earlier PBM → early intervention required
- Address PCOS- or stress-related menstrual issues
- Treat iron deficiency to improve activity tolerance

Vegetarians/vegans:

- Ensure adequate protein diversity
- Vitamin B_{12} from supplements or fortified foods

Athletes:

- *Screen for Female Athlete Triad:*
    - Low energy availability
    - Menstrual dysfunction
    - Low BMD

TAKE-HOME PEARLS

Adolescence represents the most critical window for lifelong bone health, with nearly 90% of peak bone mass achieved before adulthood. Ensuring optimal intake of calcium, vitamin D, and good quality protein during these years significantly strengthens the skeleton. Regular weight-bearing exercise and daily sunlight exposure are among the strongest modifiable determinants of bone density. At the same time, sedentary habits, carbonated drinks, restrictive diets, smoking, and early alcohol use weaken bone development and must be addressed early. Adolescents with menstrual irregularities, chronic illness, recurrent fractures, or long-term steroid use should be evaluated for low bone mass. Families, schools, and healthcare providers must work together to create supportive environments that encourage healthy eating and active living. Investing in bone health during adolescence sets the foundation for stronger bones and fewer fractures in adulthood.

MESSAGE BOX

Strong bones are built in childhood, strengthened in adolescence, and protected throughout life. Investing early is the surest way to prevent osteoporosis.

SUGGESTED READING

1. Arden NK, et al. Genetics of osteoporosis. Endocr Rev. 2005.
2. Bailey DA, et al. Peak bone mass and its importance. Bone. 1999.
3. Gammage KL, et al. Adolescents' osteoporosis knowledge. Health Educ J. 2009.
4. Gupta R, et al. Awareness about osteoporosis among adolescents. J Family Med Prim Care. 2018.

5. Harinarayan CV. Vitamin D status in India. Indian J Med Res. 2018.
6. Holick MF. Vitamin D requirements. N Engl J Med. 2007;357(3):266-81.
7. Institute of Medicine. Dietary Reference Intakes for Calcium & Vitamin D. Washington (DC): National Academies Press (US); 2011.
8. MacKelvie KJ, et al. Exercise interventions in youth. J Pediatr. 2002.
9. Marwaha RK, et al. Vitamin D status in Delhi adolescents. Indian J Pediatrics. 2011.
10. NIH Consensus Development Panel. Osteoporosis prevention, diagnosis, and therapy. JAMA. 2001;285(6):785-95.
11. Patil S, et al. Bone health awareness in Indian adolescents. Indian J Orthopedics. 2017.
12. Rizzoli R, et al. Nutrition and bone health in youth. Osteoporos Int. 2010.
13. Sheth M, et al. Effectiveness of school-based interventions. J Nutrition Education. 2012.
14. Singh P, et al. Calcium intake among adolescent girls in India. Indian J Community Med. 2019.
15. Warren MP. Role of puberty on bone health. J Clin Endocrinol Metab. 2001.
16. Weaver CM, Gordon CM, Janz KF, et al. The National Osteoporosis Foundation's position on peak bone mass development and lifestyle factors: a systematic review and implementation recommendations. Osteoporosis Int. 2016;27(4):1281-386.
17. Winzenberg T, et al. Osteoporosis education in Australian adolescents. Arch Osteoporosis. 2003.
18. Zhai F, et al. Calcium deficiency in Chinese adolescents. Asia Pac J Clin Nutr. 2005.

17 CHAPTER

Osteoporosis is Silent but Fractures are Painful—Fall and Fracture Prevention in Postmenopausal Osteoporosis

Maninder Ahuja

> *There is indeed one thing I have learnt—that an accurate diagnosis, which is relatively simple, can save women from a lot of suffering, fractures and emotional damage.*
>
> —Carmen Sanchez, osteoporosis patient from Spain, speaking at an IOF press conference held in Brussels

Osteoporosis is defined by the World Health Organization (WHO) as a "progressive systemic skeletal disease characterized by low bone mass and microarchitectural deterioration of bone tissue, with a consequent increase in bone fragility and susceptibility to fracture." Fractures in premenopausal women are less frequent than in postmenopausal women, but they may be an important indicator of underlying poor bone quality and future fracture risk.

Osteoporosis has become a major public health problem. With the acceleration of aging, the global prevalence of this disorder has reached 18.3% (Salari et al., 2021).

This is clear that osteoporosis is silent, but falls and fractures create lots of pain and misery, which kill a woman or a cause of morbidity mortality and economic burden.

Fractures occur on least trauma or fall called fragility fractures; therefor, fall preventions strategies are important.

So, let us talk about fall and fracture preventions strategies.

RISK FACTORS FOR OSTEOPOROSIS

Whenever we find risk we should be very cautious about falls and fracture prevention in these situations.

- *Gender:* Females are more prone to due to effects of sex hormones, deficiency of calcium and vitamin D and inactive lifestyle
- *Genetics*
- *Age:* The older are at higher risk of osteoporosis.
- *Peak bone mass (PBM) is the key determinant*
- *Body size:* Small, thin-boned women are at greater risk.
- *Ethnicity:* Caucasian and Asian women are at highest risk.

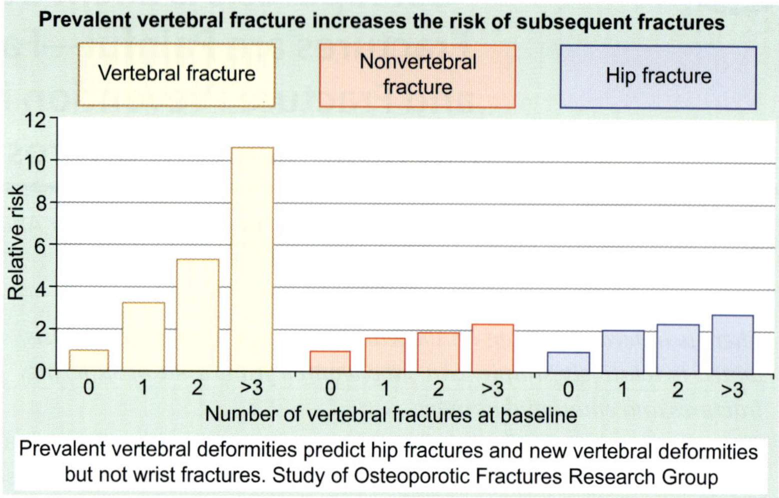

Fig. 1: First fracture increases the risk of subsequent fractures.

- *Family history*
- *Smoking*
- *Drugs:* Using steroids long-term or certain other medicines.
- *Certain diseases*, including rheumatoid arthritis, type 1 diabetes mellitus, liver disease, kidney disease, hyperthyroidism, or hyperparathyroidism
- Excessive alcohol consumption

FRAGILITY FRACTURE

- A broken bone from a slip, trip or fall from *standing height* is called a fragility fracture.
- A fragility fracture may be the first sign that our bones are weak and thin and will break easily.
- Healthy bones do not break from a simple event like a fall from standing height
- *One fracture greatly increases risk of having another one* **(Fig. 1)**

MAGNITUDE OF PROBLEM

Fractures can be devastating and may lead to: Fear (of falling, of physical activity), social isolation, depression, chronic pain, disability, hospitalization and long-term care, and even death.

Fragility fractures are a leading cause of chronic disease morbidity.

Fragility fractures are the fourth leading cause, after ischemic heart disease, dementia, and lung cancer; however, they surpass chronic obstructive pulmonary disease and ischemic stroke After sustaining a hip fracture, 10–20% of formerly community-dwelling patients require long-term nursing care. Overall, hip fractures cause the most morbidity and reported

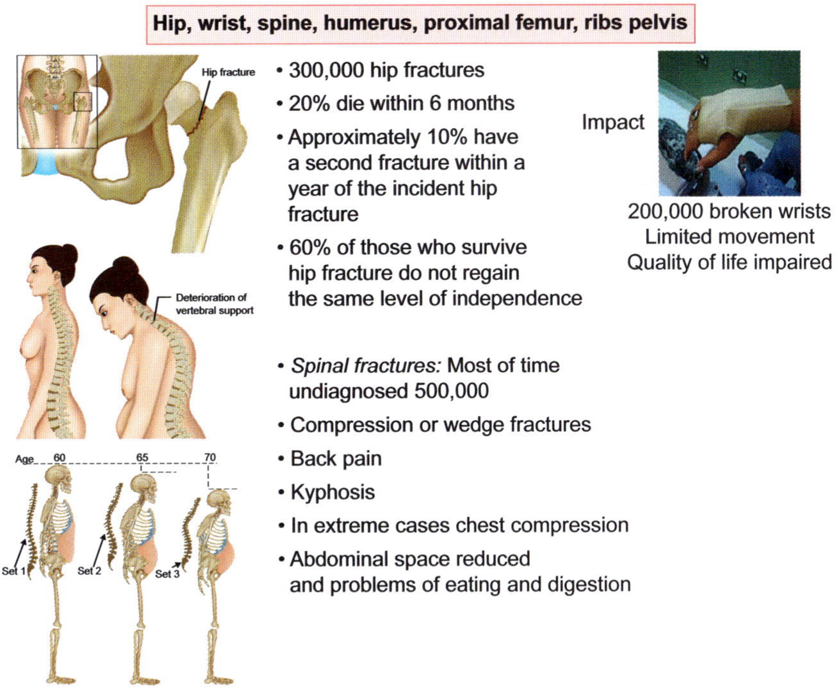

Fig. 2: Impact and extent of osteoporotic fractures.

mortality rates in up to 20–24% in the first year after a hip fracture. Loss of function and independence among survivors is profound, with 40% unable to walk independently, and 60% requiring assistance a year later **(Fig. 2)**.

PREVENTION STRATEGIES—ATTAINMENT OF PEAK BONE MASS

- First step in prevention is achievement of peak bone mass, which is important to bone health, and plays a vital part in preventing osteoporosis and subsequent fractures in later years.
- **Process of bone modeling begins during fetal growth and continues until epiphyseal fusion, usually by the end of the second decade of life. Bone modeling is sensitive to mechanical loading, emphasizing the importance of physical activity throughout growth *(Skipping and group high impact aerobic activities).***
- Bone mass is acquired relatively slowly throughout childhood. With the onset of puberty and the adolescent growth spurt in height, bone mineral accretion is rapid, reaching a peak shortly after peak gain **(Fig. 3)**.
- It is reported that hip fractures could be reduced by 30% with an increase in peak bone mass of 10%. Person who reaches peak bone mass with lower bone mineral density has less bone to lose and is more likely to develop

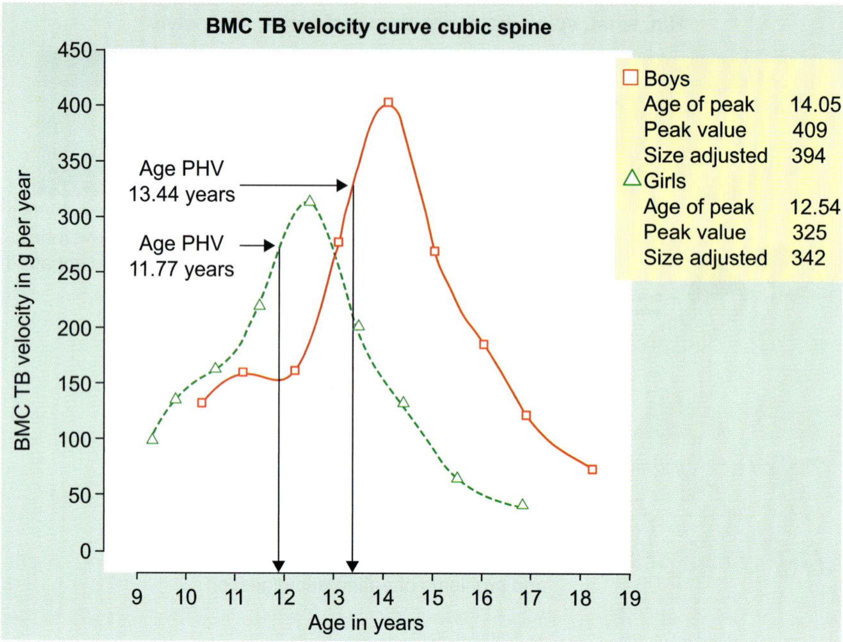

Fig. 3: BMC TB velocity curve.

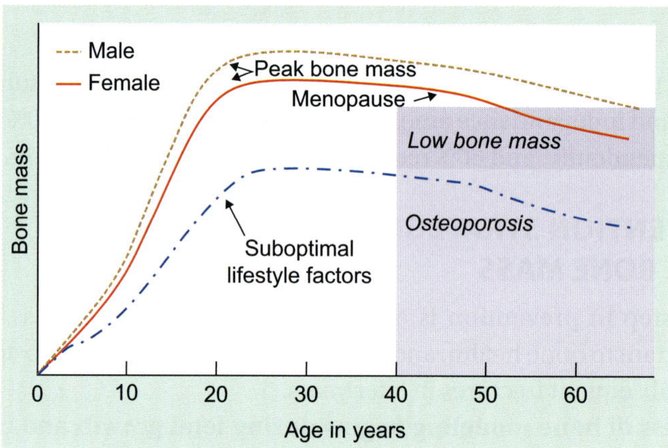

Fig. 4: Suboptimal lifestyle factors and low PBM.

osteopenia or osteoporosis sooner **(Fig. 4)**. Thus, the risk of fractures is greater and occurs earlier in life.

Fracture prevention is a multidimensional strategy:

- Attainment of PBM
- Maintenance of PBM in menopause transition
- Safe surroundings—no pot holes
- Our public places—no obstruction while walking

- Our hearing, eyes should be tested
- Reflexes should be good
- Our body protectors, when risk of fall is high
- Our body strength to be increased
- And balance exercises
- Pharmacotherapy is last height.

How body keeps balance for prevention of falls?

In *Preventing Falls*, there are two basic types of balance.

- **Static balance** gives the ability to stand up without falling over
- **Dynamic** balance allows to anticipate and react to changes as we move.

Four systems in our body work together to help stay balanced:

- **The central nervous system** coordinates movements by sending motor signals to the eyes and muscles.
- **The vestibular system** of the inner ear sends messages to the brain about the position and movements of your head in relation to the ground.
- **Vision** helps balance by showing where bodies are in relation to other objects
- **Position-sensing nerves**—called proprioceptors—embedded in muscles, tendons, and joints throughout body help move around without stumbling or bumping into things.

FALL AND FRACTURE PREVENTION EXERCISES

As we age, we are at risk of falling or tripping. This can result in broken bones or even more serious injuries because of compound effect of weak bones, weak muscles, poor hearing vision, and reflexes.

Exercising can help *prevent falls*, because it can:

- Make muscles stronger and more flexible examples squats and lunges
- Improve balance; for examples, standing erect, standing on one foot, and tandem walk
- Increase how long you can be active or maintain balance
- Adult women should engage in 150 min/week of moderate to vigorous aerobic activity exercise
- 3 days resistance training of all muscles of body should be added.

STEPS OF BALANCE

- Alignment of body **(Fig. 5)**
- Standing tall
- Standing on toes
- Standing on one foot—25 seconds
- Standing on one foot, eyes closed >6 seconds
- Walking properly and sitting properly

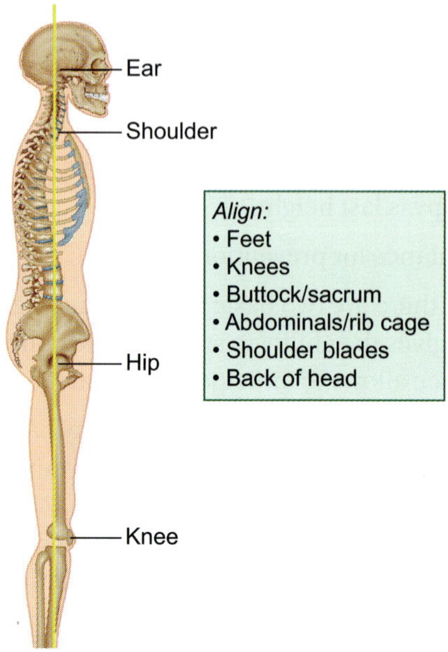

Fig. 5: Alignment of body.

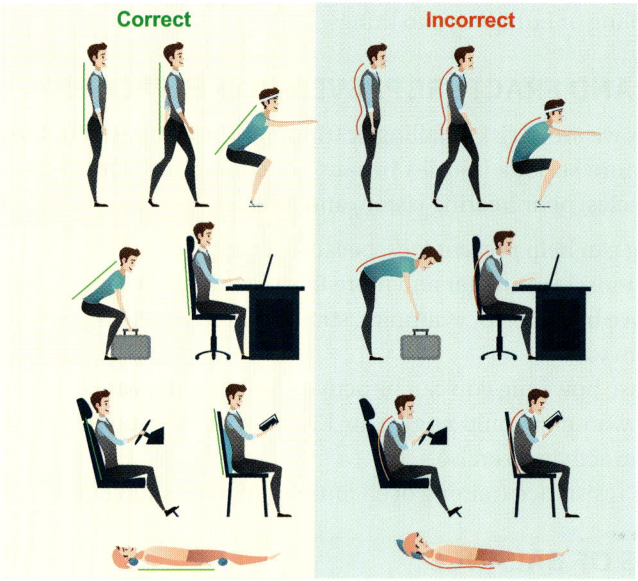

Fig. 6: Right posture.

- Take support of chair while learning
- Right posture while sitting and standing should be maintained as in **Figure 6**.

Squats with the support of a wall | Lungs with weights | Lungs without weight | Aerobic cycling

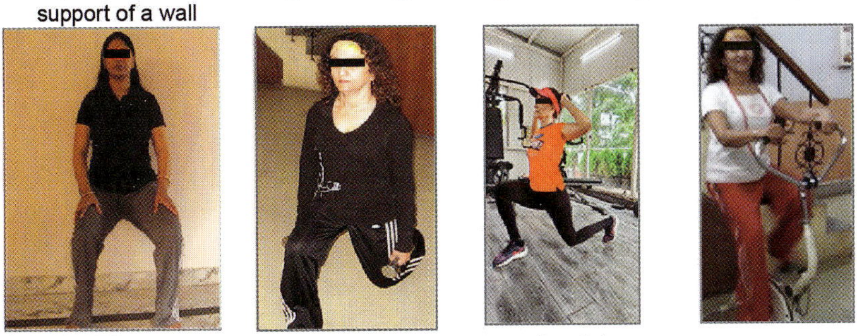

Steps of squats

1. Stand straight with feet hip-width apart. ...
2. Step 2: Engage your core muscles. ...
3. Step 3: Lower down, as if sitting in an invisible chair. ...
4. Step 4: Lift back up to standing position. ...
5. Step 5: Repeat for 10 to 15 reps, for three sets. ...

Precautions in homes

Good lighting at night, no clutter, hand rails. In bathrooms, stools for taking bath, don't lock bathroom

Fig. 7: Strengthening of muscles of legs and back.

Hip hinges to prevent spine flexion spine fractures

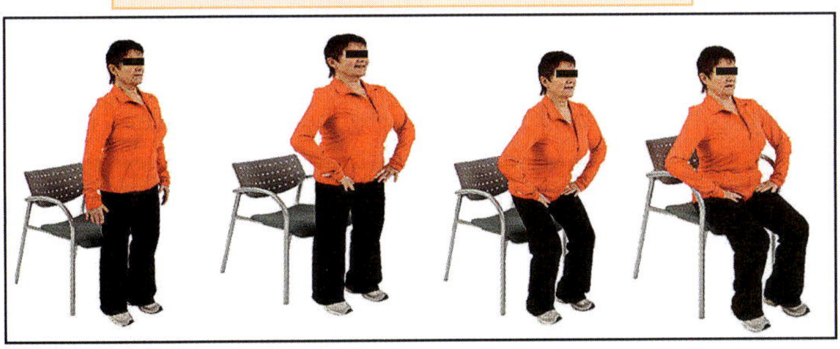

- Start with standing with good postural alignment
- Place hands in the creases of your hips
- Bend at the hips over your hands sticking your bottom out slightly and keeping back straight alignment
- Lower yourself gently onto chair keeping this alignment

When ever picking. Objects from floor don't bend your spine, bend over knees. Rotate feet and not your spine when turning

Fig. 8: Hip hinges to protect spinal.

- Strengthening of hamstrings and quadriceps—muscles of front and back of thighs is by doing squats and lunges **(Fig. 7)**.

Never bend or rotate your spine to prevent vertebral fractures, always bend on knees to pick up an object from the ground or lower level **(Fig. 8)**.

Secondary fall prevention is by pharmacological treatment of osteopenia and osteoporosis (discussed in Chapter 9). For fracture prevention, we can use orthosis **(Fig. 9)**—or supports to reduce the impact of falls.

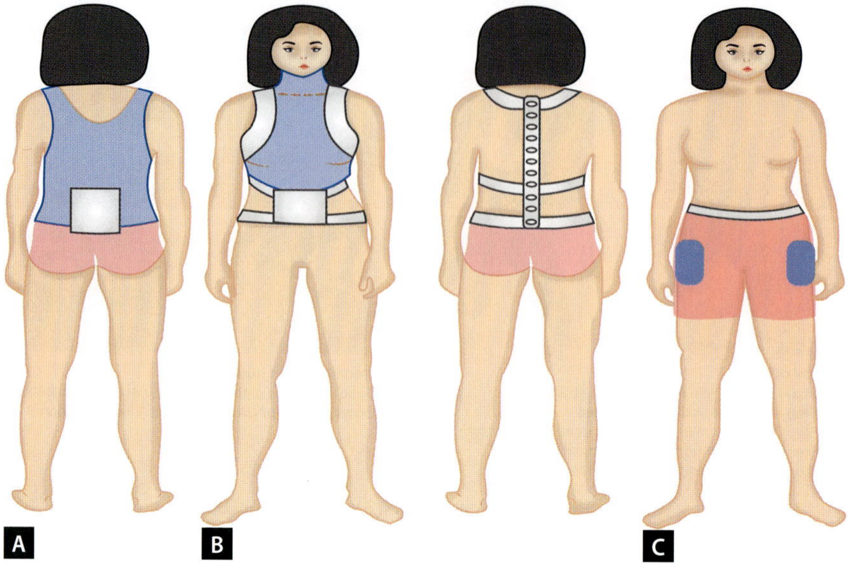

Fig. 9: Orthosis to prevent fractures by falls.

CONCLUSION

Fall prevention is an essential requirement for healthy aging and combination of strength training with balance exercises helps in fall prevention. It should be complemented by proper high protein diet and vitamin D and calcium where we need supplementation.

Regular checkup of eyesight and hearing is required along with proper lighting in the night and handrails in the bathrooms. Public places for elderly should be properly maintained with not potholes and no obstructions. Women should be advised MHT for prevention of osteoporosis and whenever required pharmacotherapy should be advised.

SUGGESTED READING

1. Consensus development conference: Diagnosis prophylaxis, and treatment of osteoporosis. Am J Med. 1993;94:646-50.
2. Sandhu SK, Hampson G. The pathogenesis, diagnosis, investigation and management of osteoporosis. J Clin Pathol. 2011;64:1042e1050.
3. Vasanwala RF, Gani L, Ang SB. It starts from the womb: maximizing bone health. Climacteric. 2022;25(1):11-21.
4. Wong RMY, Chong KC, Law SW, et al. The effectiveness of exercises on fall and fracture prevention amongst community elderlies: A systematic review and meta-analysis. J Orthopaed Trans. 2020;24.

18 CHAPTER

Role of Diet and Weight in Osteoporosis

Taruna Dua

DEFINITION

Osteoporosis is a systemic skeletal disorder characterized by low bone mineral density (BMD) and deterioration of bone microarchitecture, leading to enhanced bone fragility and an increased risk of fractures. It results from an imbalance between bone formation and bone resorption, influenced by nutritional, hormonal, metabolic, and lifestyle factors. The condition progresses silently over years, and the first clinical manifestation is often a fragility fracture of the hip, spine, or wrist.

EPIDEMIOLOGY AND SIGNIFICANCE

Osteoporosis affects millions worldwide, particularly postmenopausal women and the elderly. Nutritional intake, body weight, and lifestyle habits contribute significantly to an individual's lifetime risk. In India, widespread vitamin D deficiency, low calcium intake, and low BMI in women contribute strongly to the high prevalence of osteoporotic changes. Since bone mass achieved in early adulthood determines long-term skeletal strength, optimizing diet and weight throughout life is essential.

ROLE OF DIET IN OSTEOPOROSIS

Diet plays a foundational role in maintaining healthy bones. Nutrients influence bone remodeling, mineralization, and hormonal pathways. Key components include:

- *Calcium:*
  - Primary mineral in bone matrix.
  - Required for bone mineralization and neuromuscular function.
  - Inadequate calcium intake causes secondary hyperparathyroidism and increased bone resorption.
- *Vitamin D:*
  - Enhances intestinal absorption of calcium and phosphorus.
  - Deficiency is widespread and directly linked to low BMD.
  - Important for muscle strength and fall prevention.

- *Protein:*
  - Provides amino acids for collagen formation.
  - Essential for muscle maintenance and fracture recovery.
  - Both deficits and excessive protein may adversely affect bone; optimal intake of 0.8–1.2 g/kg/day is recommended.
- *Other micronutrients:*
  - Magnesium supports bone mineralization.
  - Vitamin K assists in activation of osteocalcin.
  - Zinc promotes osteoblast activity.
  - Potassium and antioxidants from fruits/vegetables reduce acid load and oxidative stress.

DIETARY PATTERNS AND BONE HEALTH

- *Mediterranean diet:* Rich in fruits, vegetables, nuts, and whole grains; protective due to antioxidants and anti-inflammatory effects.
- *Vegetarian diets:* Adequate if they include dairy, fortified foods, legumes, and nuts; vegan diets require careful planning to avoid deficiencies.
- *High-salt diets:* Increase urinary calcium loss.
- Excessive beverages—cola drinks, caffeine—can promote calcium excretion.

ROLE OF WEIGHT AND BODY COMPOSITION

Body weight has a direct mechanical and hormonal impact on bone. Both low and high body weight influence fracture risk differently.

- *Underweight (BMI <18.5 kg/m^2):*
  - Strong independent risk factor for osteoporosis.
  - Low mechanical loading reduces stimulus for bone formation.
  - Associated with low estrogen levels, poor nutrition, and lower vitamin D stores.
  - Common in individuals with restrictive eating patterns, chronic illness, or malabsorption.
- *Obesity and bone health:* Traditionally considered protective due to higher mechanical load, obesity is now known to have mixed effects:
  - *Benefits:* Higher load stimulates bone formation; excess adipose tissue increases estrogen production.
  - *Risks:* Visceral fat promotes inflammation, leading to bone resorption; impaired balance increases fall risk; fat infiltration into bone marrow reduces bone quality.
- *Muscle mass and bone strength:*
  - Muscle contractions apply stress on bones, stimulating remodeling.
  - Sarcopenia increases risk of falls and fractures.
  - Adequate protein and resistance exercises help preserve muscle mass.

MECHANISM: HOW DIET AND WEIGHT AFFECT BONE REMODELING

Diet affects bone metabolism through:

- Supplying minerals for bone tissue.
- Regulating hormones such as PTH and calcitonin.
- Influencing muscle strength, which stabilizes posture.

Weight affects bone metabolism through:

- Mechanical loading stimulating osteoblast activity.
- Adipose-derived hormones influencing bone turnover.
- Underweight states reducing estrogen and IGF-1, accelerating bone loss.

FLOWCHART

Adequate diet → Optimal hormonal balance + strong muscles → Balanced bone remodeling → High bone mass

Poor diet/low weight → Hormonal imbalance + weak muscles → Increased resorption → Low bone mass

CLINICAL RECOMMENDATIONS

- *Dietary advice:*
  - Ensure 1,000–1,200 mg/day calcium.
  - Maintain vitamin D level ≥30 ng/mL; supplement if needed.
  - Include high-quality protein in each meal.
  - Consume rich sources of micronutrients through fruits, vegetables, nuts, and seeds.
  - Limit processed foods, excess salt, caffeine, and carbonated drinks.
- *Weight management:*
  - Maintain BMI between 20 and 25 kg/m^2 for optimal bone density.
  - Avoid extreme dieting and rapid weight loss.
  - Encourage strength training to enhance lean mass.
- *Lifestyle modification:*
  - Weight-bearing exercises (walking, jogging, and stair climbing).
  - Balance training (yoga and, tai chi).
  - Avoid smoking and excessive alcohol.
  - Ensure adequate sun exposure.
- *Special groups:*
  - Postmenopausal women require closer dietary calcium and vitamin D monitoring.
  - Elderly individuals benefit from nutrient-dense meals and supervised exercise.
  - Adolescents should maximize peak bone mass through adequate diet and activity.

Table 1 and Figure 1 are provided separately following the main text.

TABLE 1: Role of nutrients and minerals.

Nutrient	*Function*	*Sources*
Calcium	Bone mineralization	Milk, ragi, and cheese
Vitamin D	Calcium absorption	Sunlight, eggs, and fortified foods
Protein	Collagen matrix	Pulses, legumes, and eggs
Magnesium	Bone formation	Nuts and greens
Vitamin K	Osteocalcin activation	Leafy vegetables

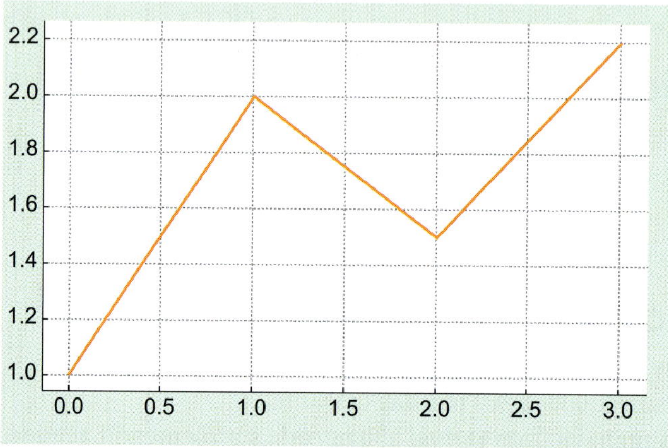

Fig. 1: Bone remodeling balance.

TAKE-HOME MESSAGES

- Diet and weight profoundly influence bone strength and fracture risk.
- Calcium, vitamin D, protein, and micronutrient-rich foods are essential for bone remodeling.
- Both underweight and obesity can adversely affect bone quality.
- Ideal BMI range of 20–25 kg/m^2 supports optimal mechanical loading.
- Muscle strength improves balance, mobility, and bone density.
- Lifestyle modification—exercise, sun exposure, smoking cessation—is crucial.
- A holistic approach combining diet, physical activity, and weight management is the most effective way to prevent osteoporosis.

SUGGESTED READING

1. Bischoff-Ferrari HA. Optimal serum 25-hydroxyvitamin D levels. Osteoporos Int. 2006;17:1519-28.
2. Bonjour JP. Nutritional approach for preventing osteoporosis. Nutr Rev. 2011;69:165-75.
3. Cashman KD. Calcium intake, calcium bioavailability and bone health. Br J Nutr. 2002;87:S169-77.
4. Compston JE, McClung MR, Leslie WD. Osteoporosis. Lancet. 2019;393:364-76.

5. Compston JE. Sex steroids and bone. Physiol Rev. 2001;81:419-47.
6. Daly RM, Bass S, Stuart AL, et al. Calcium and vitamin D supplementation on bone density. J Clin Endocrinol Metab. 2020;105:e336-45.
7. Daly RM. Exercise and bone health. Med Sport Sci. 2007;51:35-49.
8. Dawson-Hughes B. Interaction of dietary calcium and protein. Am J Clin Nutr. 2004;80:1725S-6S.
9. Eastell R, O'Neill TW, Hofbauer LC, et al. Postmenopausal osteoporosis. Nat Rev Dis Primers. 2016;2:16069.
10. Frost HM. Bone's mechanostat. Anat Rec. 1987;219:1-9.
11. Heaney RP. Functional indices of vitamin D status. Nutr Rev. 2008;66:S63-72.
12. Holick MF. Vitamin D deficiency. N Engl J Med. 2007;357:266-81.
13. Howe TE, Shea B, Dawson LJ, et al. Exercise for preventing osteoporosis. Cochrane Database Syst Rev. 2011;(7):CD000333.
14. Johnell O, Kanis JA. An estimate of worldwide prevalence of osteoporosis. J Bone Miner Res. 2006;21:487-93.
15. Kanis JA, Melton LJ, Christiansen C, et al. The diagnosis of osteoporosis. J Bone Miner Res. 1994;9(8):1137-41.
16. Lips P. Vitamin D physiology. Prog Biophys Mol Biol. 2006;92:4-8.
17. Looker AC, Melton LJ, Harris TB, et al. Prevalence of low femoral bone density. J Bone Miner Res. 1997;12:1761-8.
18. Misra M, Klibanski A. Endocrine consequences of anorexia nervosa. Lancet Diabetes Endocrinol. 2014;2:581-92.
19. Mithal A, Wahl DA, Bonjour JP, et al. Global vitamin D status and osteoporosis. Osteoporos Int. 2009;20:1807-20.
20. NIH Consensus Development Panel. Osteoporosis prevention, diagnosis, and therapy. JAMA. 2001;285:785-95.
21. Rizzoli R, Bonjour JP. Dietary protein and bone health. Osteoporos Int. 2010;21:1463-73.
22. Shapses SA, Sukumar D. Bone metabolism in obesity. Curr Opin Endocrinol Diabetes Obes. 2012;19:430-5.
23. Tucker KL. Nutrient intake and bone health. Curr Osteoporos Rep. 2009;7:111-7.
24. Weaver CM, Gordon CM, Janz KF, et al. The National Osteoporosis Foundation's position statement on peak bone mass. Osteoporos Int. 2016;27:1281-6.
25. Zhao LJ, Liu YJ, Liu PY, et al. Relationship of obesity with osteoporosis. J Clin Endocrinol Metab. 2007;92:1640-6.

19 CHAPTER

Clinical Diagnosis of Osteoporosis in OPD

Shubhi Gupta, Neelam Aggarwal

INTRODUCTION

Osteoporosis is a progressive systemic skeletal disorder characterized by low bone mass and microarchitectural deterioration of bone tissue, ultimately leading to enhanced bone fragility and an increased risk of fractures. It is widely recognized as a major global public health problem, particularly affecting postmenopausal women and the elderly population. With the rise in life expectancy, the burden of osteoporosis-related morbidity, disability, and healthcare expenditure continues to increase worldwide.

Clinically, osteoporosis is often termed a "silent disease" because individuals typically remain asymptomatic until the first fragility fracture occurs. These fractures, especially of the hip, vertebrae, and distal radius, not only impair quality of life but are also associated with increased mortality. Therefore, early clinical diagnosis plays a crucial role in preventing complications, guiding timely therapeutic interventions, and reducing long-term disability.

The diagnosis of osteoporosis traditionally relies on bone mineral density (BMD) assessment using dual-energy X-ray absorptiometry (DXA), which remains the gold standard. According to the World Health Organization (WHO) criteria, a T-score ≤ –2.5 at the lumbar spine, total hip, or femoral neck is diagnostic of osteoporosis. However, clinical assessment extends beyond BMD alone, as many fragility fractures occur in individuals with T-scores in the osteopenic range. Thus, it is essential to combine BMD findings with clinical risk factors, detailed history, physical examination, and tools such as the FRAX fracture risk calculator to achieve a comprehensive diagnosis.

Furthermore, identifying secondary causes of osteoporosis—including endocrine disorders, malabsorption syndromes, chronic inflammatory diseases, and long-term glucocorticoid therapy—is vital for appropriate management. Effective clinical diagnosis in OPD settings requires a structured, point-wise approach using flowcharts, tables, and risk-evaluation pathways to ensure accuracy, efficiency, and reproducibility.

Early detection and comprehensive diagnosis remain the cornerstone for preventing osteoporotic fractures and improving patient outcomes.

RISK FACTORS FOR OSTEOPOROSIS

- *Nonmodifiable:*
  - Age >50 years
  - Female sex
  - Postmenopausal status
  - Family history of fragility fractures
  - Low BMI (<19 kg/m^2)
- *Modifiable:*
  - Sedentary lifestyle
  - Smoking, alcohol use
  - Low calcium and vitamin D intake
  - Prolonged immobilization
  - Poor nutrition
- *Secondary causes:*
  - *Endocrine:* Hyperthyroidism and Cushing's syndrome
  - *Malabsorption:* Celiac disease
  - *Drugs:* Steroids, anticonvulsants, and heparin

CLINICAL ASSESSMENT IN OPD

- *History:*
  - Previous fragility fractures
  - Height loss >2 cm
  - Menstrual/menopause history
  - Chronic diseases affecting bone health
  - Medication review
- *Physical examination:*
  - Kyphosis
  - Reduced height
  - Gait imbalance
  - Bone tenderness
  - Historical height loss (>6 cm)
  - Measured height loss (<2 cm)
  - Significant height loss should be investigated by a lateral thoracic and lumbar spine X-ray.

Clinical assessment of osteoporosis in the OPD setting focuses on identifying high-risk individuals early through a structured evaluation. A detailed medical history is the first essential step, emphasizing prior fragility fractures, premature menopause, chronic illnesses, long-term glucocorticoid use, height loss, and family history of hip or vertebral fractures. Assessment of lifestyle risk factors—dietary calcium deficiency, low physical activity, smoking, and alcohol consumption—is equally important.

TABLE 1: Recommendations for clinical assessment.

Assessment	*Recommendations for clinical assessment recommended elements of clinical assessment*	
Physical examination	• Measure weight (weight loss of ≥10% since age 25 is significant)	
	• Measure height annually (prospective loss >2 cm) • (historical height loss >6 cm) • Measure rib to pelvis distance ≤2 fingers' breadth • Measure occiput-to-wall distance far (for kyphosis) >5 cm	Diagnosis of vertebral fractures
	• Assess fall risk by using Get-Up-and-Go Test (ability to get out of chair without using arms, walk several steps and return)	

Physical examination should aim to detect clinical signs of vertebral fractures such as kyphosis, loss of height, and tenderness over the spine. Measurement of height at every visit is valuable, as a reduction >2 cm may indicate vertebral compression. Gait imbalance or muscle weakness may further increase fall risk **(Table 1)**.

After clinical assessment, patients with significant risk factors should undergo targeted evaluation for secondary causes including endocrine disorders, malabsorption, chronic inflammatory states, and renal dysfunction. This is followed by BMD measurement using DXA, supported by fracture prediction tools like FRAX. A well-structured point-wise OPD assessment improves diagnostic accuracy and ensures timely intervention to prevent fractures.

DIAGNOSTIC APPROACH (FLOWCHART 1)

Flowchart 1: Clinical diagnosis of osteoporosis.

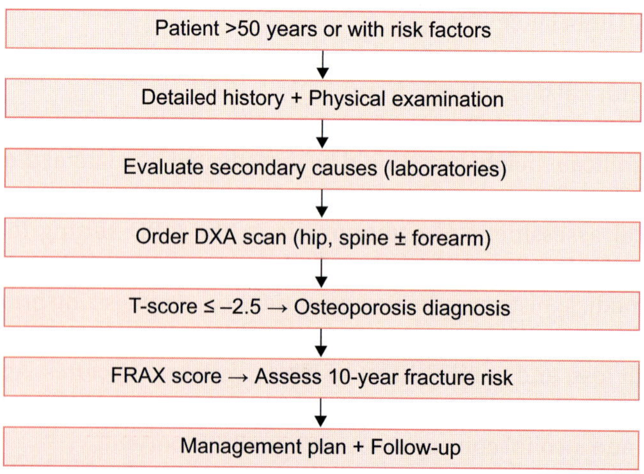

INVESTIGATIONS

Investigations for osteoporosis aim to confirm low bone mineral density, identify secondary causes, and assess fracture risk. The primary diagnostic tool is DXA, which measures BMD at the lumbar spine, total hip, and femoral neck, with forearm DXA reserved for cases where hip or spine evaluation is not feasible. DXA provides the T-score, interpreted using WHO criteria to classify normal bone density, osteopenia, or osteoporosis.

Basic laboratory evaluation is essential to rule out secondary osteoporosis. Recommended baseline tests include serum calcium, phosphorus, alkaline phosphatase, 25-hydroxy vitamin D, complete blood count, renal and liver function tests. These help detect common metabolic abnormalities such as vitamin D deficiency, renal impairment, or high bone turnover.

Further targeted investigations are advised when history or clinical findings suggest specific secondary causes. These include thyroid-stimulating hormone (TSH) for hyperthyroidism, parathyroid hormone (PTH) for hyperparathyroidism, serum cortisol for Cushing's syndrome, and celiac screening for malabsorption. In men, serum testosterone may be required to identify hypogonadism.

Additional imaging such as VFA or spine X-rays may be used in patients with height loss or back pain to detect asymptomatic vertebral fractures.

A comprehensive investigation approach enables accurate diagnosis and guides individualized treatment.

BONE MINERAL DENSITY TESTING

- *Gold standard:* Dual-energy X-ray absorptiometry
- *Sites:* Lumbar spine, total hip, femoral neck, and forearm (if spine/hip not measurable)
- *Interpretation (WHO criteria):* Normal: T-score ≥ –1, Osteopenia: –1 to –2.5, Osteoporosis: ≤ –2.5, Severe Osteoporosis: ≤ –2.5 + fragility fracture

LABORATORY EVALUATION

- *Basic tests:*
  - CBC
  - ESR
  - Serum calcium
  - Phosphorus
  - ALP
  - 25(OH) Vitamin D
  - Renal and liver functions
- *Secondary causes:*
  - TSH
  - PTH

- Serum cortisol
- Celiac panel
- Testosterone (men)

CLINICAL TOOLS FOR DIAGNOSIS

- *FRAX tool:*
  - Evaluates 10-year probability of major osteoporotic and hip fracture
  - Uses age, sex, BMI, prior fracture, smoking, glucocorticoids, etc.
- *QUS (quantitative ultrasound):*
  - Useful screening tool in low-resource OPD
  - Not used for monitoring therapy

IMAGING

Imaging plays a vital role in the diagnosis of osteoporosis, detection of fragility fractures, and assessment of structural bone changes. While BMD is measured using DXA, additional imaging modalities help identify fractures that may be clinically silent.

Dual-energy X-ray Absorptiometry

Dual-energy X-ray absorptiometry is the gold standard for measuring BMD at the lumbar spine, total hip, and femoral neck. It provides T-scores that classify normal bone density, osteopenia, and osteoporosis. DXA also offers VFA, a low-radiation lateral spine image that helps detect previously unrecognized vertebral compression fractures.

Conventional Radiography (X-rays)

Plain X-rays of the thoracolumbar spine are useful in identifying vertebral compression fractures, wedge deformities, endplate changes, and reduced trabecular patterns. However, X-rays detect bone loss only after 30–40% of mineral content has been lost, limiting their sensitivity.

Vertebral Fracture Assessment

Vertebral fracture assessment performed on DXA machines provides rapid, low-dose imaging for vertebral morphology assessment. It is particularly useful in older adults, patients with height loss >2 cm, chronic back pain, or long-term steroid use.

Other Imaging

In selected cases, MRI may be required to differentiate acute from chronic fractures, while CT helps evaluate complex vertebral deformities or atypical femoral fractures.

TABLE 2: Major risk factors for osteoporosis.

Nonmodifiable	*Modifiable*	*Secondary causes*
• Age • Female sex • Menopause • Family history	• Smoking • Alcohol • Low calcium intake • Inactivity	• Endocrine disorders • Drugs (steroids) • Malabsorption

Imaging, combined with clinical findings and BMD, provides a comprehensive diagnostic approach.

Table 2 shows risk factors for osteoporosis.

TAKE-HOME MESSAGES

- Osteoporosis is often silent until fracture, requiring proactive clinical diagnosis.
- A combination of history, physical examination, risk factor assessment, and laboratory evaluation is essential in OPD practice.
- DXA scan remains the gold standard for diagnosis, using WHO T-score criteria.
- FRAX tool provides essential fracture risk prediction and guides treatment initiation.
- Always rule out secondary causes through targeted laboratory tests, especially in younger patients.
- Utilize flowcharts, tables, and point-wise assessment for rapid decision-making in busy clinical settings.
- Identify vertebral fractures early using X-ray or VFA, even in asymptomatic patients.
- Use SI units, standard abbreviations, and generic drug names.

SUGGESTED READING

1. Blake GM, Fogelman I. The role of DXA bone density scans in the diagnosis and treatment of osteoporosis. Bone. 2013;55(1):7-19.
2. Compston J, Cooper A, Cooper C, et al. UK clinical guideline for the prevention and treatment of osteoporosis. Lancet. 2019;393(10169):364-76.
3. Cummings SR, Melton LJ. Epidemiology and outcomes of osteoporotic fractures. JAMA. 2002;288(15):1889-97.
4. Genant HK, Wu CY, van Kuijk C, et al. Vertebral fracture assessment using imaging. J Bone Miner Res. 1993;8(9):1137-48.
5. Haentjens P, Magaziner J, Colon-Emeric C, et al. Meta-analysis: excess mortality after hip fracture among older women and men. J Bone Miner Res. 2010;25(10):1436-44.
6. Heaney RP. Calcium, dairy products and osteoporosis. J Am Coll Nutr. 2000;19(2):715-21.
7. Holick MF. Vitamin D deficiency. N Engl J Med. 2007;357(3):266-81.
8. Johnell O, Kanis JA. An estimate of the worldwide prevalence and disability associated with osteoporotic fractures. Osteoporos Int. 2006;17(12):1726-33.
9. Kanis JA, Melton LJ, Christiansen C, et al. The diagnosis of osteoporosis. Osteoporos Int. 2005;16(4):498-500.
10. Kanis JA, Oden A, Johansson H, et al. FRAX and its applications to clinical practice. Osteoporos Int. 2008;19(6):385-97.

11. Kanis JA, on behalf of the World Health Organization Scientific Group. Assessment of osteoporosis and fracture risk. Osteoporos Int. 2008;19(4):385-97.
12. Krieg MA, Barkmann R, Gonnelli S, et al. Quantitative ultrasound in the management of osteoporosis. Osteoporos Int. 2008;19(6):777-88.
13. Lane NE. Epidemiology, etiology, and diagnosis of osteoporosis. Ann Intern Med. 2006;144(9):734-40.
14. Lewiecki EM. Benefits and limitations of vertebral fracture assessment (VFA). Osteoporos Int. 2010;21(3):441-6.
15. Siris ES, Chen YT, Abbott TA, et al. Bone mineral density thresholds for pharmacological intervention to prevent fractures. Arch Intern Med. 2004;164(10):1108-12.
16. Watts NB, Bilezikian JP, Camacho PM, et al. American Association of Clinical Endocrinologists medical guidelines for clinical practice for the diagnosis and treatment of postmenopausal osteoporosis. J Clin Endocrinol Metab. 2010;95(6):211-38.
17. WHO Scientific Group. Assessment of osteoporosis at the primary health-care level. WHO Press. 2007;5:1-85.
18. World Health Organization. Assessment of fracture risk and its application to screening for postmenopausal osteoporosis: report of a WHO Study Group. World Health Organ Tech Rep Ser. 2003;843:1-129.

CHAPTER 20

Pharmacological Management of Osteoporosis

Mayank Vashishtha, Ajay Aggarwal, Aakansha Shukla, Setu Gupta

PHARMACOTHERAPY OF OSTEOPOROSIS

INTRODUCTION

Osteoporosis is a systemic skeletal disorder characterized by low bone mass and microarchitectural deterioration of bone tissue, which increases bone fragility and fracture risk. It is a silent disease that causes fractures in the hip, vertebrae, and wrist.

DEFINITION

Osteoporosis is defined by the World Health Organization (WHO) as Bone mineral density (BMD) T-score ≤ -2.5 SD at hip or spine using dual-energy X-ray absorptiometry (DXA scan).

EPIDEMIOLOGY

- *Global prevalence:* Approximately 200 million individuals.
- One-third of postmenopausal women are affected.
- One in every five men over the age of 50 years is affected.
- Increased fracture-related morbidity and mortality pose a significant burden on the aging population.

PATHOPHYSIOLOGY

- Bone remodeling requires a balance of osteoclastic bone resorption and osteoblastic bone formation.
- Postmenopausal osteoporosis is caused by an estrogen deficiency. Increase RANKL and osteoclast activity.
- Senile osteoporosis is characterized by decreased osteoblast function and low vitamin D levels.
- Secondary causes include glucocorticoids, endocrine disorders, and chronic systemic diseases.

PHARMACOLOGY GOALS

- Prevent fractures in the hip, vertebrae, and wrist.
- Improve BMD by stabilizing or increasing bone mass.

- Improve bone quality. Improve the architecture.
- Reduce morbidity and mortality while improving quality of life.

INDICATIONS FOR PHARMACOTHERAPY

Patients with any of the following should begin treatment:

- T-score ≤ –2.5 in the femoral neck or lumbar spine
- History of fragility fractures.
- A T-score of –1.0 to –2.5 indicates osteoporosis, with a 10-year FRAX risk of ≥20% (>10% for India) for major osteoporotic fracture or ≥3% for hip fracture.
- Long-term glucocorticoid use (≥5 mg prednisolone daily for over 3 months).

CLASSIFICATION (TABLE 1)

Bisphosphonates

Mechanism of Action

- Inhibit osteoclast-mediated bone resorption, thereby reducing bone turnover.
- Result in increased bone mineral density and reduced fracture risk.

TABLE 1: Classification.

Category	*Drugs*
Antiresorptive agents	Bisphosphonates, denosumab, SERMs, hormone therapy, and calcitonin
Anabolic agents	Teriparatide, abaloparatide, and romosozumab
Others	Vitamin D and calcium supplements

TABLE 2: Pharmacological agents in osteoporosis.

Drug	*Route*	*Standard dose*	*Frequency*	*Typical duration*
Alendronate	Oral	70 mg	Once weekly	3–5 years
Risedronate	Oral	35 mg weekly/ 150 mg monthly	Weekly or monthly	3–5 years
Ibandronate	Oral	150 mg	Once monthly	3–5 years
	IV	3 mg	Every 3 months	3–5 years
Zoledronic acid	IV	5 mg	Once yearly	3 years (postmenopausal), up to 6 years in high-risk patients

Adverse Effects

- *Gastrointestinal:* Gastric irritation, dyspepsia, esophagitis, and esophageal ulceration. Oral drugs needs to be consumed on empty stomach, and the patient needs to remain upright for at least 30–45 minutes to prevent the reflux.
- *Skeletal:* Osteonecrosis of the jaw (rare), atypical femoral shaft fractures with long-term use.
- *Acute phase reaction:* Flu-like symptoms, fever (especially with IV administration).
- Hypocalcemia (more common in renal impairment or vitamin D deficiency).

Contraindications

- Severe renal impairment (eGFR <30 mL/min for most agents; <35 mL/min for alendronate).
- Esophageal motility disorders (achalasia, strictures, and Barrett's esophagus).
- Hypocalcemia or untreated vitamin D deficiency.
- Pregnancy and lactation.

Denosumab

Mechanism of Action

Fully human monoclonal antibody targeting RANKL, thereby inhibiting osteoclast differentiation, function, and survival.

Dose: 60 mg subcutaneously every 6 months

Risks/adverse effects: Hypocalcemia, increased infection risk, and significant rebound bone loss with risk of multiple vertebral fractures upon abrupt discontinuation

Key point: Upon stopping denosumab, transition to a bisphosphonate is essential to prevent rapid bone turnover and rebound fractures.

SERMs (Selective Estrogen Receptor Modulators)

Raloxifene

- *Mechanism of action:* Estrogen agonist on bone, antagonist on breast/uterus
- Decrease vertebral fracture, increase DVT risk
- Useful in women with breast cancer risk
- Does NOT reduce hip fracture risk.

Hormone Replacement Therapy

- *Drugs:* Estrogen and estrogen-progesterone
- *Indications:* <60 years postmenopausal women with vasomotor symptoms, or the patient is within 10 years of onset of menopause, patients should be at a low risk of DVT and are not at an increased risk of breast cancer or cardiovascular diseases.
- *Benefits:* Maintains bone density
- *Risks:* Breast cancer and thromboembolism

Calcitonin

- *Mechanism:* Inhibits osteoclast activity
- *Use:* Short-term pain relief in acute vertebral fractures
- *Route:* Nasal spray or injection (not first-line therapy)

ANABOLIC THERAPY

Teriparatide and Abaloparatide

- *Mechanism of action:* Recombinant PTH (1–34)—stimulates osteoblasts → bone formation
- Used for severe osteoporosis, multiple fractures, and failure of antiresorptives
- *Dose:* 20 µg SC daily (maximum 24 months)
- *Benefits:* Decrease vertebral and nonvertebral fractures
- Risks of hypercalcemia and leg cramps and primary hyperparathyroidism needs to be ruled out before starting the therapy.

Romosozumab

- *Mechanism of action:* Antisclerostin antibody (dual action)—increase formation and decrease resorption
- *Dose:* 210 mg monthly SC for 12 months
- Best for very high-risk cases, multiple fractures
- *Caution:* Cardiovascular risk (avoid in MI and stroke patients)

ADJUNCTIVE THERAPY

- Calcium and Vitamin D
- Calcium: 1,200 mg/day (diet + supplements)
- Vitamin D: 800–1,000 IU/day
- Correct vitamin D deficiency before initiating antiresorptive therapy.
- Vitamin D enhances calcium absorption and prevents hypocalcemia.

MONITORING AND FOLLOW-UP

- *BMD (DEXA):* Every 1–2 years
- *Serum calcium and vitamin D:* Every 6–12 months
- *Renal function (for bisphosphonates):* Before each IV dose

KEY POINTS

- Osteoporosis is a silent systemic skeletal disorder leading to bone fragility and fractures.
- Pharmacotherapy aims to prevent fractures, improve quality of life, and enhance bone strength.
- Drugs are categorized as antiresorptive (bisphosphonates, denosumab, and SERMs) and anabolic agents (teriparatide, abaloparatide, and romosozumab).
- Bisphosphonates remain first line due to efficacy and cost-effectiveness.
- Denosumab is useful in renal impairment and bisphosphonate-intolerant patients.
- Anabolic agents are reserved for severe or refractory cases.
- Adequate calcium and vitamin D supplementation is essential with all therapies.
- Drug choice depends on fracture risk, comorbidities, cost, and patient characteristics.
- Monitoring includes BMD, vitamin D, calcium, and renal function.
- Combination and sequential therapy may optimize long-term outcomes.

SUGGESTED READING

1. Assessment of fracture risk and its application to screening for postmenopausal osteoporosis. Report of a WHO Study Group. World Health Organ Tech Rep Ser. 1994;843:1-129.
2. Black DM, Rosen CJ. Clinical Practice. Postmenopausal Osteoporosis. N Engl J Med. 2016;374(3):254-62. Erratum in: N Engl J Med. 2016;374(18):1797.
3. Borgström F, Karlsson L, Ortsäter G, et al.; International Osteoporosis Foundation. Fragility fractures in Europe: burden, management and opportunities. Arch Osteoporos. 2020;15(1):59.
4. Chesnut CH 3rd. Treatment of postmenopausal osteoporosis. Compr Ther. 1984;10(7):41-7.
5. Compston JE, McClung MR, Leslie WD. Osteoporosis. Lancet. 2019;393 (10169):364-76.
6. Cosman F, Crittenden DB, Adachi JD, et al. Romosozumab Treatment in Postmenopausal Women with Osteoporosis. N Engl J Med. 2016;375(16):1532-43.
7. Cummings SR, Eckert S, Krueger KA, et al. The effect of raloxifene on risk of breast cancer in postmenopausal women: results from the MORE randomized trial. Multiple Outcomes of Raloxifene Evaluation. JAMA. 1999;281(23):2189-97.
8. de Villiers TJ, Pines A, Panay N, et al.; International Menopause Society. Updated 2013 International Menopause Society recommendations on menopausal hormone therapy and preventive strategies for midlife health. Climacteric. 2013;16(3):316-37.
9. Eastell R, Rosen CJ, Black DM, et al. Pharmacological Management of Osteoporosis in Postmenopausal Women: An Endocrine Society* Clinical Practice Guideline. J Clin Endocrinol Metab. 2019;104(5):1595-622.

10. Holick MF. Vitamin D deficiency. N Engl J Med. 2007;357(3):266-81.
11. Kanis JA, Johnell O, Oden A, et al. FRAX and the assessment of fracture probability in men and women from the UK. Osteoporos Int. 2008;19(4):385-97.
12. Miller PD, Wagman RB, Peacock M, et al. Effect of denosumab on bone mineral density and biochemical markers of bone turnover: six-year results of a phase 2 clinical trial. J Clin Endocrinol Metab. 2011;96(2):394-402.
13. Neer RM, Arnaud CD, Zanchetta JR, et al. Effect of parathyroid hormone (1-34) on fractures and bone mineral density in postmenopausal women with osteoporosis. N Engl J Med. 2001;344(19):1434-41.
14. Saag KG. Glucocorticoids in chronic disease: The good, the bad, the bone. Trans Am Clin Climatol Assoc. 2023;133:69-80.
15. Weaver CM, Alexander DD, Boushey CJ, et al. Calcium plus vitamin D supplementation and risk of fractures: an updated meta-analysis from the National Osteoporosis Foundation. Osteoporos Int. 2016;27(1):367-76. Erratum in: Osteoporos Int. 2016;27(8):2643-6.

21 CHAPTER

Osteoporosis Challenges and Future Directions

Archana Dwivedi, Saraswathi Kondapalli

INTRODUCTION

Osteoporosis is a systemic skeletal disorder characterized by reduced bone strength and deterioration of bone micro architecture, leading to increased fracture risk. It affects over 200 million women globally and remains one of the most under diagnosed and undertreated chronic diseases in women's health. Although osteoporosis occurs in both sexes, women experience a significantly higher burden due to hormonal changes, lower peak bone mass, and longer life expectancy. As populations age worldwide, the prevalence of osteoporotic fractures—especially hip, vertebral, and wrist fractures—is rising, placing substantial physical, emotional, and financial strain on women and healthcare systems.

This chapter highlights major challenges in prevention, diagnosis, and management of osteoporosis in women, and outlines future directions that could transform care.

EPIDEMIOLOGICAL BURDEN IN WOMEN

The menopausal transition is a critical period for bone health. Nearly 20–30% of lifetime bone loss occurs in the first 5–7 years after menopause due to estrogen deficiency. Hip fractures in postmenopausal women carry a one-year mortality rate of up to 20%, and many survivors experience long-term disability and dependence. Vertebral fractures, though often clinically silent, lead to chronic pain, kyphosis, impaired lung capacity, and reduced quality of life.

TABLE 1: Risk factors for osteoporosis.

Category	*Risk factors*
Nonmodifiable	Female sex, age >50 years, early menopause, family history, and low BMI
Modifiable	Smoking, alcohol, sedentary lifestyle, and low sun exposure
Nutritional	Low calcium, vitamin D deficiency, and low protein
Medical/drug-related	Hyperthyroidism, RA, CKD, and steroids

With increasing longevity, osteoporosis is becoming one of the most significant noncommunicable conditions affecting healthy aging in women.

CHALLENGES IN OSTEOPOROSIS DIAGNOSIS

Under Diagnosis and Late Detection

Osteoporosis is frequently diagnosed only after the first fragility fracture. Many women remain unaware of their bone health status due to the asymptomatic nature of the disease. Even among high-risk postmenopausal women, screening rates are suboptimal.

Limited Access to BMD Testing

Dual-energy X-ray absorptiometry (DXA) is the gold standard for diagnosis, yet access remains limited in low-resource regions. Cost, lack of awareness, and limited availability restrict timely assessment.

Limitations of Risk Assessment Tools

The FRAX® algorithm is widely used to predict fracture risk, but it does not fully incorporate fall risk, bone quality, or cortical porosity. Studies show that falls predict fractures independently of FRAX probability, highlighting the need for improved tools.

Emerging adjuncts like Trabecular Bone Score (TBS) and AI-enhanced imaging may offer better risk stratification but are not yet universally accessible.

Overreliance on T-scores

Many fractures occur in women classified with osteopenia rather than osteoporosis by DXA criteria, suggesting that diagnostic thresholds may overlook women at high fracture risk.

TABLE 2: Investigations in osteoporosis.

Investigation	*Purpose*
DXA	Gold standard diagnosis
Serum calcium/phosphate	Detect metabolic disorders
25(OH) Vitamin D	Check deficiency
TSH	Rule out hyperthyroidism
PTH	Detect hyperparathyroidism
Renal function	Before bisphosphonate use
BTMs (P1NP, CTX)	Assess treatment response

CHALLENGES IN PREVENTION

Inadequate Calcium and Vitamin D Intake

Many women fail to meet recommended calcium and vitamin D intakes due to dietary patterns, limited sun exposure, and cultural practices. Vitamin D deficiency is particularly widespread in South Asia and the Middle East.

Poor Awareness Across Life Stages

Most educational efforts target older women, even though adolescence is critical for achieving peak bone mass. Pregnancy, lactation, and perimenopause require targeted counseling, yet awareness remains limited.

TABLE 3: Key challenges in osteoporosis management.

Challenge	*Description*	*Impact*
Underdiagnosis	Often undetected until fragility fracture	Higher morbidity and mortality
Low awareness	Patients underestimate risk; fear therapy	Low adherence
Limited DXA access	Machines concentrated in cities	Delayed diagnosis
Adherence issues	GI intolerance; fear of side effects	Reduced treatment impact
Secondary causes missed	Thyroid, CKD, steroids	Persistent bone loss
Falls not addressed	Lack of balance training	More fractures
Long-term therapy gaps	Bisphosphonate holidays; denosumab rebound	Clinical confusion

TABLE 4: Treatment options and limitations.

Drug class	*Examples*	*Advantages*	*Limitations*
Bisphosphonates	Alendronate, Zoledronate	Strong evidence	GI effects, ONJ
SERMs	Raloxifene	Vertebral fracture reduction	VTE risk
Hormone therapy	Estrogen ± Progesterone	Effective early postmenopause	VTE and cancer risk
Denosumab	RANKL inhibitor	Potent antiresorptive	Rebound fractures
Anabolics	Teriparatide	Rapid bone formation	Cost, duration limit
Romosozumab	Sclerostin inhibitor	Dual action	Cardiovascular concerns

Physical Inactivity

Sedentary lifestyles significantly reduce mechanical stimulation essential for bone formation. Weight-bearing activities are proven to maintain bone health but are not practiced consistently by many women.

Sociocultural Barriers

Dietary restrictions, body image concerns, and limited prioritization of women's health in some regions contribute to inadequate preventive care.

CHALLENGES IN TREATMENT

Low Treatment Initiation and Poor Adherence

Even after diagnosis, treatment rates remain low. Many women discontinue medications within 1–2 years due to fears of side effects or misconceptions about therapy duration.

Safety Concerns with Long-term Therapy

Bisphosphonates are effective but associated with rare complications such as atypical femoral fractures and osteonecrosis of the jaw. Denosumab discontinuation can result in rebound vertebral fractures unless followed by appropriate transition therapy.

Limited Access to Advanced Therapies

Anabolic agents like teriparatide and romosozumab demonstrate substantial reductions in fractures but are costly and often not covered by insurance, limiting access for women in many countries.

Lack of Fracture Liaison Services

Fracture liaison services (FLS) programs identify fracture patients early, ensure DXA evaluation, initiate treatment, and track adherence. Despite proven effectiveness, FLS remains underdeveloped in many regions.

MENOPAUSE AND OSTEOPOROSIS: A CRITICAL INTERSECTION

Estrogen deficiency accelerates bone turnover, with osteoclast activity exceeding osteoblast capacity. Hormone replacement therapy (HRT) is effective for preventing bone loss in early postmenopausal women, but concerns about cardiovascular and cancer risks have drastically reduced its use. Updated guidelines emphasize individualized risk-benefit assessment, especially in women under 60 or within 10 years of menopause onset.

Special Populations at Risk

Premature Ovarian Insufficiency (POI)

Women with POI have earlier and more severe estrogen deficiency, placing them at very high lifetime risk of osteoporosis. Lifelong hormone therapy is often required.

Women with Chronic Medical Conditions

Rheumatoid arthritis, thyroid disorders, diabetes, celiac disease, and chronic liver disease all compromise bone health. Steroid-induced osteoporosis is particularly common among women treated for autoimmune diseases.

Post-bariatric Surgery Women

Rapid weight loss and nutrient malabsorption significantly accelerate bone loss after bariatric surgery. These women require intensive monitoring and supplementation.

Psychosocial and Economic Challenges

Impact on Quality of Life

Vertebral fractures cause chronic pain, disability, height loss, and psychological distress. Many women experience depression and social isolation due to fear of falling.

Economic Burden

Healthcare costs of osteoporotic fractures—including hospitalization, surgery, and rehabilitation—are considerable. The indirect burden on caregivers and families is particularly great for older women who lose independence.

FUTURE DIRECTIONS

Mechanism-based Screening and Early Detection

AI-Assisted Imaging

AI algorithms applied to routine radiographs can detect early structural deterioration, enabling opportunistic screening.

TABLE 5: Future directions in osteoporosis.

Area	*Development*	*Expected benefit*
Novel drugs	Cathepsin K inhibitors	More effective therapy
Personalized medicine	Genomic profiling	Tailored care
Digital health	Fall detection tech	Reduced fractures
Advanced screening	AI-enhanced DXA	Early detection
Bone regeneration	Stem cells	True bone rebuilding

Assessing Bone Quality

Advanced tools like high-resolution peripheral quantitative CT (HR-pQCT) and bone turnover markers improve fracture prediction beyond BMD alone.

Personalized and Genomic Medicine

Emerging genetic markers (e.g., COL1A1 and LRP5 variants) may enable early identification of women at high risk. Machine learning incorporating genetics, lifestyle, and imaging may enable precision therapy.

Advancements in Pharmacotherapy

Novel Anabolic Agents

Romosozumab represents a major advance with dual effects—stimulating bone formation and reducing resorption. More such molecules are under development.

Long-acting Depot Formulations

Future therapies may involve annual or biannual injections, improving adherence.

Safe Transition Protocols

New evidence is emerging on how to manage denosumab discontinuation to prevent rebound fractures.

Regenerative Medicine

Stem cell therapies, osteoinductive scaffolds, and 3D bioprinting offer future potential for regenerating osteoporotic bone. Although currently experimental, they may revolutionize treatment for severe osteoporosis.

Digital Technologies and Fall Prevention

Wearable devices and smartphone-based gait analysis can detect balance issues early. AI-driven fall prediction models may help prevent fractures in older women.

Strengthening Health Policy

Key policy improvements include:

- Integrating osteoporosis screening into routine women's health programs
- Vitamin D fortification
- Community exercise programs
- Insurance support for anabolic therapies
- Nationwide implementation of FLS programs

CONCLUSION

Osteoporosis remains a major threat to women's health, with challenges spanning prevention, diagnosis, treatment adherence, and access to care. However, rapid advances in imaging, pharmacotherapy, regenerative science, and digital health provide exciting opportunities for better outcomes. A proactive, multidisciplinary approach, coupled with stronger health policies, is essential to reduce the burden of fractures and ensure a healthier future for women worldwide.

SUGGESTED READING

1. Bilezikian JP, Lewiecki EM, Miller PD, McClung MR. Osteoporos Int. 2016;27:1917-8.
2. Black DM, Rosen CJ. Postmenopausal Osteoporosis. N Engl J Med. 2016;374:254-62.
3. Compston J, Cooper A, Cooper C, et al. UK clinical guideline for the prevention and treatment of osteoporosis. Arch Osteoporos. 2017;12(1):43.
4. Cosman F, de Beur SJ, LeBoff M, et al. Clinician's Guide to Prevention and Treatment of Osteoporosis. Osteoporos Int. 2014;25:2359-81.
5. Eastell R, Rosen CJ, Black DM, et al. Lancet Diabetes Endocrinol. 2019;7:901-21.
6. Ensrud KE, Crandall CJ. Osteoporosis. Ann Intern Med. 2017;167(3):ITC17–ITC32.
7. Harvey NC, Odén A, Orwoll E, et al. Osteoporos Int. 2018;29:1831-40.
8. Johnell O, Kanis JA. Osteoporos Int. An estimate of the worldwide prevalence and disability associated with osteoporotic fractures. 2006;17:1726-33.
9. Kanis JA, Cooper C, Rizzoli R, Reginster JY. European guidance for the diagnosis and management of osteoporosis in postmenopausal women. Osteoporos Int. 2019;30(1):3-44.
10. Kanis JA, Harvey NC, McCloskey E, et al. Algorithm for the management of patients at low, high and very high risk of osteoporotic fractures. Osteoporos Int. 2020;31:1-12.
11. Lane JM, Russell L, Khan SN. Osteoporosis. Clin Orthop Relat Res. 2000;(372):139-50.
12. McClung MR, Grauer A, Boonen S, et al. Romosozumab in postmenopausal women with low bone mineral density. N Engl J Med. 2014;370:412-20.
13. NIH Consensus Development Panel. Osteoporosis prevention, diagnosis, and therapy. JAMA. 2001;285:785-95.
14. Paschalis EP, Shane E, Lyritis G, et al. Bone fragility and collagen cross-links. J Bone Miner Res. 2004;19(12):2000-4.
15. Rachner TD, Khosla S, Hofbauer LC. Osteoporosis: now and the future. Lancet. 2011;377:1276-87.
16. Reid IR, Bolland MJ, Grey A. Effects of vitamin D supplements on bone mineral density: a systematic review and meta-analysis. Lancet. 2014;383(9912):146-55.
17. Riggs BL, Khosla S, Melton LJ. Sex steroids and the construction and conservation of the adult skeleton. Endocr Rev. 2002;23:279-302.
18. U.S. Preventive Services Task Force. Screening for osteoporosis: U.S. Preventive Services Task Force recommendation statement. Ann Intern Med. 2011;154:356-64.
19. Watts NB, Adler RA, Bilezikian JP, et al. Osteoporosis in men: an Endocrine Society clinical practice guideline. J Clin Endocrinol Metab. 2012;97(6):1802-22.
20. WHO Scientific Group. Assessment of osteoporosis at the primary healthcare level. WHO; 2007.

22 CHAPTER

Role of Exercise and Type of Exercise for Osteoporosis

Manju Varma

INTRODUCTION

Osteoporosis is a progressive systemic skeletal disease characterized by reduced bone mass, compromised bone strength, and microarchitectural deterioration of bone tissue, resulting in increased bone fragility and heightened susceptibility to fracture.

The global burden of osteoporosis is substantial and growing. An estimated 2.7 million hip fractures occur worldwide annually, with approximately 75% affecting women.

Osteoporosis is a metabolic bone disease that progress silently leading to loss of bone mass. The fractures caused because of osteoporotic bones are widely prevalent in India and are one of the common causes of morbidity and mortality in elderly population. The health care providers and physiotherapist have a specific role in osteoporosis through exercise prescription, education and strategies to maximize function, reduce the risk of falls and manage pain. There are various treatment protocols involved in the treatment and prevention of osteoporosis, among which the exercises have an impact on the bone mineral density.

Osteoporosis is commonly managed medically and typically with treatment. Exercise is also essential in the management of osteoporosis but tends to be underutilized due to lack of knowledge and unfounded concerns about the risk of injury. In fact, optimal care of people with low bone mass, osteoporosis and/or increased risk of falling can and should include targeted exercise to help prevent osteoporotic fracture.

Osteoporosis statistics in India show a prevalence of about 18.3%, which is higher in women (19.4%) and elderly (37.0%) one in five adults have osteoporosis and almost one in two has osteopenia. Around six crore people are affected, the majority being women, nearly one out three is postmenopausal

The risk of breaking the bone is one out of two women aged > 50 years.

Exercises for osteoporosis are the best form of prevention and treatment. Many exercises can be performed by anyone, no matter their age or fitness level.

Osteoporosis is a condition where a person's bones lose calcium and other minerals, which makes them fragile (breaking). According to a research study, osteoporosis and fragility fractures are an expensive human and socioeconomic burden everywhere in the world.

Even with osteoporosis, it is never too late to begin a bone-healthy exercise program. One may be concerned that being active increases the chances of falling and breaking a bone. However, the opposite is true.

A regular, well-designed exercise program may aid in the prevention of falls and fractures. This is because exercise strengthens bones and muscles while improving balance, coordination, and flexibility. This is critical for people who have osteoporosis.

THE ADVANTAGES OF EXERCISE FOR PEOPLE WHO HAVE OSTEOPOROSIS

Fractures are more likely to occur when sedentism, poor posture, balance, and weak muscles are present. Numerous approaches, including exercise, can help persons with osteoporosis improve their health. Other benefits include:

- Reduction in bone loss
- Increased physical fitness since the residual bone tissue is preserved.
- Strengthened muscles
- Enhanced reaction time and increased mobility
- Improved coordination and balance
- Decreased chance of bone fractures brought on by falls
- Pain relief, increased vigor, and better mood

EXERCISE COMPONENTS

Before starting a new exercise regimen, consult with the doctor and physical therapist. They can advise what is safe the level of exercise, overall health, and stage of osteoporosis.

There is not a single fitness program that works for everyone with osteoporosis. the routine should depend on one's age, the severity of osteoporosis, and the medication one is taking right now.

Additional medical diseases such as arthritis, cardiovascular or pulmonary illness, and neurological issues affect one's ability and fitness.

Improving bone density or preventing falls should be the major objectives of one exercise regimen. Mix specific balance exercises with weight-bearing aerobic and muscle-building (resistance) training is preferable.

Exercises Recommended for Osteoporosis

- Weight-bearing/impact
- Resistance/strengthening
- Posture
- Balance
- Flexibility
- Functional activities

Exercising with weights: One should do them on the feet, which forces the bones and muscles to work against gravity to keep one upright. the bones respond to weight by strengthening and building themselves.

Weight-bearing *exercise is classified into two types:* High-impact and low-impact.

1. *High impact exercises:* Dancing, high-impact aerobics, hiking, jogging/running, jumping rope, stair climbing, tennis, volleyball
2. *Low-impact exercises:* Elliptical training machines, stair-step machines, low-impact aerobics, walking on a treadmill, walking on level surfaces.

Resistance exercise: It is the best way to strengthen bone and muscle with dumbbells and barbells, elastic band resistance, body-weight resistance, or weight-training machines.

Tai chi and other posture, balance, and body strength exercises:

- *Posture exercises*
  Posture is critical in all activities.
  These exercises improve posture and reduce rounded or "sloping" shoulders. They can help to decrease the risk of breaking a bone, especially in the spine.
  Corner Stretch
- *Hip and back (spine) strengthening exercises*
  These exercises can help to strengthen the muscles in the back and hips.
  Hip Abductor Strengthening, Prone Leg Lifts
- *Balance exercises*
  Decrease fall risk.
  These exercises strengthen legs and challenge the balance. They can decrease the chance of falling.
  Toe Raises/Heel Raises, Wall Slide
- *Functional exercises*

These exercises improve how well one move. They can help in everyday activities and decrease the chance of falling and breaking a bone. For example, if one find it hard to get up from a chair or climb stairs, one should do these activities as exercises (try standing up and sitting down several times until you are tired).

Exercises/Activities People with Osteoporosis Avoid

A person who has osteoporosis has weakened bones that are prone to breaking. They should avoid engaging in activities such as:

- Forward spine flexion with weighted loads, such as abdominal sit-ups. Increases the likelihood of one falling. It needs quick, strong action unless taught gradually as part of a progressive program.
- A powerful twisting motion, like a golf swing, is necessary unless the person is accustomed to such movements.
    - Undue compressive strain on the spine
    - Rotation with excess loading
    - High risk movement patterns
    - High impact work
    - High intensity training at outset
    - Emphasize good technique, especially neutral spine
    - Carefully consider program design
    - Consider other pathology

Contraindications to Exercise

Absence of any of the following:

- Unstable angina
- Uncompensated congestive heart failure
- Severe aortic stenosis
- Uncontrolled arrhythmias
- Severe pain
- Uncontrolled blood pressure
- Untreated medical causes of falls, e.g., syncopal/blackout episodes.

Recommendations for the Frequency and Duration of Exercise

The precise amount of exercise required for people with osteoporosis is unknown. However, guidelines recommend:

- 45 minutes to 1 hour of aerobic exercise twice or three times a week
- Each resistance training session should include exercises to develop the lower limb, trunk, and arm muscles. Resistance training should be done twice or three times a week. 8–10 times should be given to each exercise.
- Exercises to improve the balance should be done twice a week for a few minutes at a difficult level. For safety reasons, always ensure to have something one can grip on if one overbalance something.
- Exercises that promote flexibility include stretching.

One must consistently perform the activities throughout time to lower the risk of suffering a bone fracture.

OTHER THINGS ONE CAN DO TO IMPROVE BONE HEALTH

- Exercise is an essential component of any osteoporosis treatment plan.
- Before beginning a new exercise program, consult with the doctor. Expert advice can be obtained from physiotherapists and other exercise professionals.
- Always begin the exercise program at a low level and gradually progress.
- Exercising too quickly and vigorously may increase the risk of injury, including fractures.
- Also, talk to the rheumatologist or dietitian about ways to boost the calcium, vitamin D, and other essential nutrient intakes. They may suggest to take supplements. Smoking and excessive alcohol consumption are both terrible for the bones.
- Exercising for osteoporosis is a significant part of managing the condition, and one should start working on it as soon as possible.

TAKE-HOME MESSAGES

No matter what is the age or the state of bone health, regular exercise will be beneficial.

- Set achievable goals-and then gradually and progressively advance in difficulty.
- Warm up (for example, stretching) before exercise and listen to the body. Some muscle soreness after exercise is normal, sharp pain is not.
- Find types of physical activity one enjoys—that way one will be more likely to continue in the long term.
- If one has fragile bones due to osteoporosis or there is a history of fall, it is a good idea to consult a physiotherapist who can help plan a targeted, safe and effective exercise program.

SUGGESTED READING

1. Birge SJ, Dalsky G. The role of exercise in preventing osteoporosis. CDC Stacks; 1989.
2. Camacho PM, Petak SM, Binkley N, et al. American associations of clinical endocrinologists/American college of endocrinology clinical practice guidelines for the diagnosis and treatment of postmenopausal osteoporosis----2020 update. Endocr Pract. 2020;26(Suppl 1):1-46.
3. Cussler EC, Lohman TG, Going SB, et al. Weight lifted in strength training predicts bone change in postmenopausal women. Med Sci Sports Exerc. 2003;35(1):10-7.
4. Gerontologia Polska. 2016;24:214-18.
5. Hartley A, Gregson CL, Hannam K, et al Sarcopenia is negatively related to high gravitational impacts achieved from day-to-day physical activity. J Gerontol Ser A Biol Sci Med Sci. 2018;73(5):652-9.
6. Hartley GW, Roach KE, Nithman RW, et al. Physical Therapist Management of Patients With Suspected or Confirmed Osteoporosis: A Clinical Practice Guideline From the Academy of Geriatric Physical Therapy. J Geriatr Phys Ther. 2022;44(2):E103-E119.
7. Kelley GA, Kelley KS, Tran ZV, et al. Resistance training and bone mineral density in women; a meta-analysis of controlled trials. Am J Phys Med Rehabil. 2001;80(1):65-77.

8. Lange U, Teichman J, Uhlemann C. Current knowledge about physiotherapeutic strategies in osteoporosis prevention and treatment. Rheumatol Int. 2005;26:99-106.
9. Lindsey C, et al. Evaluation for the effect of exercise on posture, back strength, pain. Papper Presented at: WCPT: Washington; 1995.
10. Sinaki M. Journal fur Mineralstoffwechsel & Muskuloskelettale Erkrankungen. 2010;17(2):62-5.
11. Wolfson L, Whipple R, Derby C, et al. Balance and strength training in older adults: intervention gains and Tai Chi Maintenance. J Am Geriatr Soc. 1996;44(5):498-506.

23 CHAPTER

Osteoporosis in Postmenopausal Women and Its Diagnostic Evaluation with DEXA Scan/BMD (Bone Mineral Density)

SS Doda

INTRODUCTION

Osteoporosis is a long-standing disease in which bones become fragile due to loss of minerals/calcium and are more likely to break. If not prevented or left untreated, osteoporosis can progress painlessly until a bone breaks. These fractures often occur in the hip, spine or wrist. Whereas, osteopenia is having a bone density, lower than normal. Osteoporosis may remain a silent disease for long time. It increases your risk of bone fractures. Bone fractures are usually painful. Common fractures sites include fractures of the vertebrae, hip and forearm bones. Fractured vertebrae can also cause a loss of height and a curved spine.

The osteoporotic patients have decreased bone density and fragile bones, meaning these bones can break even with trivial trauma. There is increased incidence of reduced bone density/osteopenia/Osteoporosis with advancing age, particularly in postmenopausal women.

The risk factors include:

- Advanced age
- Menopause
- Low calcium diet
- Family history of osteoporosis
- Eating disorders
- History of previous bone fracture
- Thin body frame
- Caucasian or Asian ethnicity
- Hyperthyroidism (overactive thyroid) and diabetes
- Certain medicines (such as steroids, anticonvulsants and anti-cancer treatment)
- High caffeine intake
- Females (especially when early menopause and/or removal of the ovaries has occurred)
- Low testosterone level in males.

Some lifestyle factors that increase chance of getting osteoporosis are:

- Smoking
- Drinking excessive amount of alcohol
- Not moving around and exercising enough-low physical activity
- Not getting enough calcium, vitamin D and protein in your diet

DIAGNOSIS OF OSTEOPOROSIS/OSTEOPENIA

Bone is lost with ageing and declining estrogen and testosterone levels, particularly after menopause in women. Advanced age, prior fragility fracture and low T scores less than –2.5 are the greatest risks factors for fractures. DEXA (dual energy X-ray absorptiometry) is considered the diagnostic modality of choice for measuring bone mineral density. In younger postmenopausal women, guidelines recommend DEXA only in those who have a substantial risk of fracture based on clinical factors.

DEXA Scan

- DEXA was first commercially introduced in 1987.
- The principle includes two X-ray beams with two different energy peaks (70 kV and 140 kV) passing through the body, one gets absorbed by the soft tissues and the other by the bones.
- Soft tissue amount is subtracted from the total area, giving the bone mineral density.
- Data is fed into computer powered with a complex algorithm to calculate BMD values.
- These measurements are then compared with the normal ranges matched for chronological age (T and Z scores).

DEXA Procedure

The scanner continuously samples the bone mineral content (BMC) as it moves in a rectilinear pattern over the areas of the region of interest. The resulting series of transverse profiles provides the data base for quantitative analysis.

The quantities estimated by DEXA are:

- Area, expressed in cm^2, which is the 2-D projection of the bone.
- Bone mineral content (BMC) is expressed in grams.
- Bone mineral density (BMD) is expressed in g/cm^2
- BMD results are reported in g/cm^2, and T score is the difference, in standard deviations, between the patient's value and the mean value for healthy 30 year old of the same sex and Z score is the difference between the patient's value and the mean value of people of same age, race and sex.

- The clinical purpose of a DEXA scan is to screen patients for low bone mass and osteoporosis and also help estimate fracture risk.

DEXA Sites

DEXA scan is usually performed for:

- *Central:* Lumbar spine, hip, whole body
- *Peripheral:* Forearm, calcaneum
- *Lumbar spine:* Measures BMD from L1 to L4 and compiles scores
- *Hip:* Measures BMD from femoral neck, trochanter and intertrochanter region and compiles scores.

Indications for DEXA Scan

- Women >65 years
- Men >70 years
- Postmenopausal women and men > 50 years, based on risk factor profile.

Recommendations

The National Osteoporosis Foundation and the International Society of Clinical Densitometry both recommend DEXA for postmenopausal women under age 65 years. Those in the menopausal transition who have clinical risk factors for fracture such as:

- Low body weight
- History of prior fracture
- A disease or condition associated with bone loss
- Use of medications that cause bone loss such as steroids.
  DEXA is also recommended in women to monitor treatment response.

Contraindications for DEXA

- Pregnancy
- Recent administration of contrast or radio-nuclide scan
- Radio opaque implant in measurement area
- Marked obesity

Interpretation of DEXA Results

What are T and Z Scores?

The T-score is calculated by taking the difference between a patient's measured BMD and the mean BMD of the young normal population matched for gender and ethnicity, and then by dividing the difference with the standard deviation (SD) of the BMD of the young normal population.

$$\text{T-score} = \frac{\text{Patient's measured BMD} - \text{Mean BMD of young normal population}}{\text{SD of BMD of young normal population}}$$

TABLE 1: WHO interpretation of t score results.

T-Score	*% of bone loss*
0.0	0
–1.0	10%
–2.0	20%
–2.5	25%
–3.0	30%
–4.0	40%

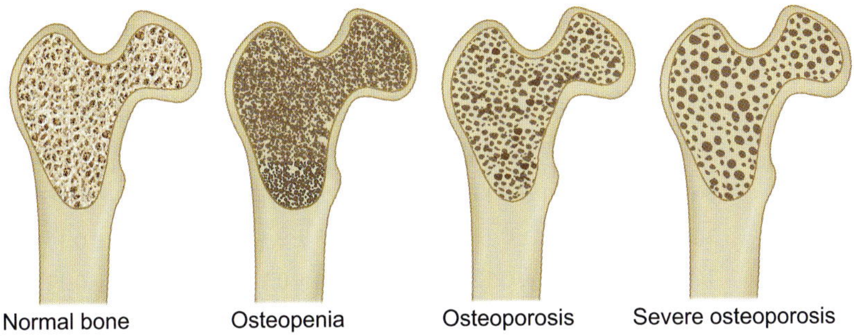

Fig. 1: Stages of osteoporosis.

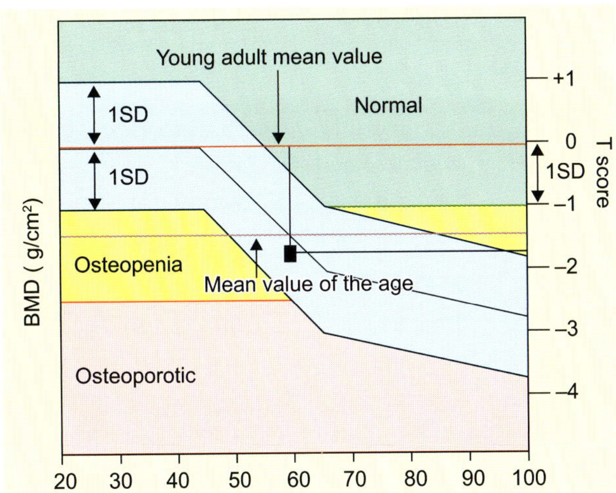

Fig. 2: Bone density assessment by WHO.

A 10% loss of bone mass (equivalent to a 1 standard deviation decrease in the T score) in the vertebrae can double the risk of vertebral fractures.

A 10% loss of bone mass in the hip can cause a 2.5 times greater risk of hip fracture.

Z-SCORE

The Z-score compares your results to a person of same gender and age as yourself. In other words, the Z-score is calculated, comparing a patient to age-matched group

$$\text{Z-score} = \frac{\text{Patient's measured BMD–Mean BMD of age-matched group}}{\text{SD of BMD of age-matched group}}$$

A Z-score less than –2.0 indicates low bone mass

TABLE 2: BMD expressed in g/cm^2 (males).

Age (years)	*Number*	*Lumbar spine 1–4*	*Total hip*	*Femoral neck*
10–89	7,837	0.945 ± 0.154	0.954 ± 0.134	0.803 ± 0.138
50–89	3,314	0.938 ± 0.156	0.920 ± 0.130	0.742 ± 0.122
10–19	902	0.797 ± 0.167	0.899 ± 0.146	0.808 ± 0.148
20–29	865	1.001 ± 0.115	1.025 ± 0.122	0.916 ± 0.167
30–39	1,351	0.991 ± 0.118	0.993 ± 0.116	0.854 ± 0.118
40–49	1,405	0.975 ± 0.126	0.988 ± 0.118	0.823 ± 0.115
50–59	1,221	0.955 ± 0.141	0.976 ± 0.117	0.791 ± 0.113
60–69	1,174	0.943 ± 0.155	0.926 ± 0.122	0.745 ± 0.112
70–79	773	0.914 ± 0.174	0.862 ± 0.123	0.683 ± 0.110
80–89	146	0.887 ± 0.164	0.797 ± 0.138	0.630 ± 0.121

TABLE 3: BMD expressed in g/cm^2 (females).

Age (years)	*Number*	*Lumbar spine 1–4*	*Total hip*	*Femoral neck*
10–89	9,368	0.893 ± 0.159	0.840 ± 0.131	0.699 ± 0.129
50–89	3,849	0.791 ± 0.139	0.764 ± 0.119	0.613 ± 0.108
10–19	821	0.845 ± 0.146	0.847 ± 0.121	0.738 ± 0.121
20–29	1,086	0.962 ± 0.107	0.890 ± 0.104	0.775 ± 0.104
30–39	1,794	0.995 ± 0.115	0.896 ± 0.106	0.760 ± 0.103
40–49	1,818	0.989 ± 0.122	0.913 ± 0.109	0.759 ± 0.103
50–59	1,267	0.858 ± 0.131	0.838 ± 0.104	0.684 ± 0.098
60–69	1,369	0.787 ± 0.123	0.769 ± 0.098	0.615 ± 0.087
70–79	988	0.733 ± 0.132	0.696 ± 0.101	0.548 ± 0.087
80–89	225	0.691 ± 0.122	0.625 ± 0.096	0.489 ± 0.081

PATIENT BIOGRAPHICAL:

Name:					
Patient ID:		**Birth Date:**	01-Mar-42	**Height:**	161.0 cm
Gender:	Female	**Exam Date:**	05-Dec-22	**Weight:**	60.0 kg
Indications:		**Fractures:**		**Treatments:**	

ASSESSMENT:

The BMD measured at AP Spine L1-L4 is 1.369 g/cm² with a T-score of 1.6. This patient is considered normal according to World Health Organization (WHO) criteria. Fracture risk is low.

The BMD measured at Femur Neck Left is 0.919 g/cm² with a T-score of -0.9. Bone density is up to 10% below young normal. This patient is considered normal according to World Health Organization (WHO) criteria. Fracture risk is low.

The BMD measured at Femur Neck Right is 0.980 g/cm² with a T-score of -0.4. Bone density is up to 10% below young normal. This patient is considered normal according to World Health Organization (WHO) criteria. Fracture risk is low.

The BMD measured at Femur Total Left is 0.986 g/cm² with a T-score of -0.2. Bone density is up to 10% below young normal. This patient is considered normal according to World Health Organization (WHO) criteria. Fracture risk is low.

The BMD measured at Femur Total Right is 1.004 g/cm² with a T-score of 0.0. This patient is considered normal according to World Health Organization (WHO) criteria. Fracture risk is low.

Site	Region	Measured Date	Measured Age	WHO Classification	Young Adult T-score	BMD
AP Spine	L1-L4	05-Dec-22	80.7	Normal	1.6	1.369 g/cm²
DualFemur	Neck Left	05-Dec-22	80.7	Normal	-0.9	0.919 g/cm²
DualFemur	Neck Right	05-Dec-22	80.7	Normal	-0.4	0.980 g/cm²
DualFemur	Total Left	05-Dec-22	80.7	Normal	-0.2	0.986 g/cm²
DualFemur	Total Right	05-Dec-22	80.7	Normal	0.0	1.004 g/cm²

World Health Organization (WHO) criteria for post-menopausal, Caucasian Women:
Normal: T-score at or above -1 SD
Osteopenia: T-score between -1 and -2.5 SD
Osteoporosis: T-score at or below -2.5 SD

FOLLOW-UP:

People with diagnosed cases of osteoporosis or at high risk for fracture should have regular bone mineral density tests. For patients eligible for Medicare, routine testing is allowed once every 2 years. The testing frequency can be increased to one year for patients who have rapidly progressing disease, those who are receiving or discontinuing medical therapy to restore bone mass, or have additional risk factors.

Based on these results, a follow-up exam is recommended in December 2024

CONSULTANT RADIOLOGIST

Fig. 3: Normal DEXA report of a patient, 80 years, female (Page 1).

Birth Date:	01-Mar-42 80.7 years	**Referring Physician:**			
Height / Weight:	161.0 cm 60.0 kg	**Measured:**	05-Dec-22	10:43:03 AM	(14.10)
Sex / Ethnic:	Female Asian	**Analyzed:**	08-Dec-22	6:22:08 PM	(14.10)

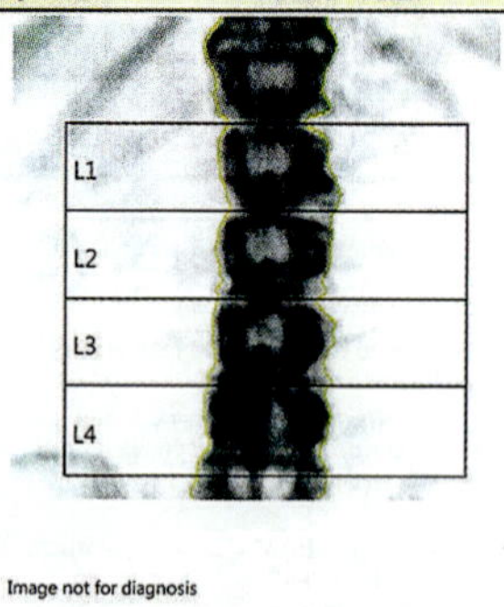

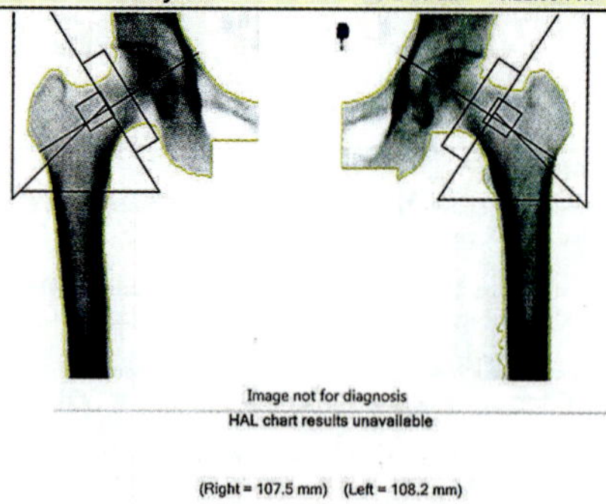

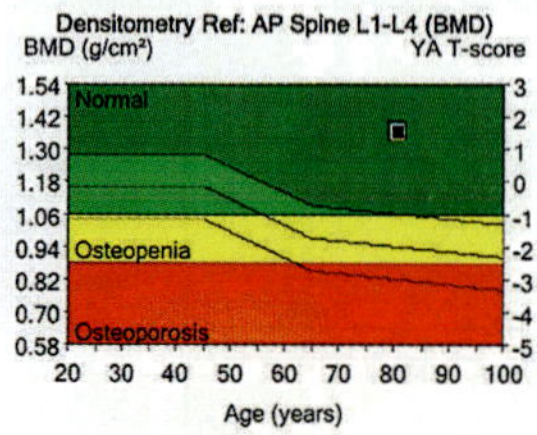

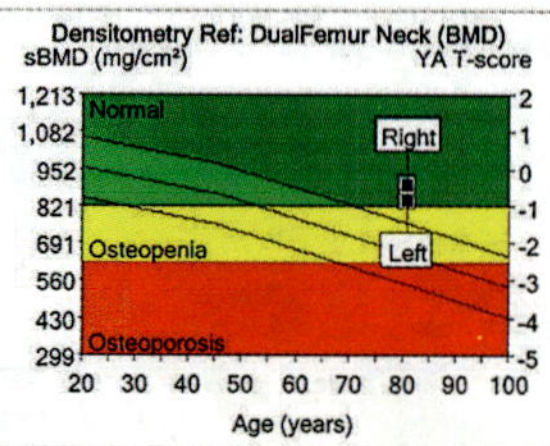

Region	sBMD[1] (mg/cm²)	Young-Adult[2,7] T-score	Age-Matched[3] Z-score	WHO Classification[11]
AP Spine L1-L4	-	1.6	3.6	Normal
DualFemur Neck				
Left	840	-0.9	1.4	Normal
Right	897	-0.4	1.9	Normal
Mean	869	-0.6	1.7	Normal
Difference	57	0.4	0.4	-

1 - Statistically 68% of repeat scans fall within 1SD (± 0.010 g/cm² for AP Spine L1-L4); (± 13 mg/cm² for DualFemur Neck Left)
2 - USA (Combined NHANES (ages 20-30) / Lunar (ages 20-40)) AP Spine Reference Population (v113); USA (Combined NHANES (ages 20-30) / Lunar (ages 20-40)) Femur Reference Population (v113)
3 - AP Spine Matched for Age, Weight (females 25-100 kg), Ethnic; DualFemur Matched for Age, Weight (females 25-100 kg), Ethnic
7 - DualFemur Total T-score difference is 0.1. Asymmetry is None.
11 - World Health Organization - Definition of Osteoporosis and Osteopenia for Caucasian Women: Normal = T-score at or above -1.0 SD; Osteopenia = T-score between -1.0 and -2.5 SD; Osteoporosis = T-score at or below -2.5 SD; (WHO definitions only apply when a young healthy Caucasian Women reference database is used to determine T-scores.)

Fig. 4: Normal DEXA Report of a patient, 80 years, female (Page 2).

Birth Date:	01-Mar-42	80.7 years	**Referring Physician:**			
Height / Weight:	161.0 cm	60.0 kg	**Measured:**	05-Dec-22	10:43:03 AM	(14.10)
Sex / Ethnic:	Female	Asian	**Analyzed:**	08-Dec-22	6:23:54 PM	(14.10)

ANCILLARY RESULTS

Region	BMD[1] (g/cm²)	sBMD (mg/cm²)	Young-Adult[2] (%)	T-score	Age-Matched[3] (%)	Z-score	BMC (g)	Area (cm²)	Width (cm)	Height (cm)
L1	1.258	-	111	1.1	142	3.1	15.65	12.44	3.9	3.15
L2	1.316	-	110	1.0	137	3.0	16.70	12.69	4.0	3.15
L3	1.456	-	121	2.1	152	4.1	17.37	11.93	4.2	2.85
L4	1.509	-	126	2.6	157	4.6	19.03	12.62	4.4	2.84
L1-L2	1.287	-	111	1.0	139	3.0	32.35	25.13	4.0	6.30
L1-L3	1.342	-	115	1.4	145	3.4	49.72	37.05	4.1	9.15
L1-L4	1.384	-	117	1.7	147	3.7	68.75	49.67	4.2	11.99
L2-L3	1.384	-	115	1.5	144	3.5	34.07	24.62	4.1	6.00
L2-L4	1.426	1,358	119	1.9	149	3.9	53.10	37.23	4.2	8.83
L3-L4	1.483	-	124	2.4	155	4.4	36.40	24.55	4.3	5.68

1 - Statistically 68% of repeat scans fall within 1SD (± 0.010 g/cm² for AP Spine L1-L4)
2 - USA (Combined NHANES (ages 20-30) / Lunar (ages 20-40)) AP Spine Reference Population (v113)
3 - Matched for Age, Weight (females 25-100 kg), Ethnic
Filename: vqjemr6img.dfx

Fig. 5: Normal DEXA report of a patient, 80 years, female (Page 3).

Birth Date:	01-Mar-42 80.7 years	**Referring Physician:**	
Height / Weight:	161.0 cm 60.0 kg	**Measured:**	05-Dec-22 10:45:21 AM (14.10)
Sex / Ethnic:	Female Asian	**Analyzed:**	05-Dec-22 10:45:37 AM (14.10)

ANCILLARY RESULTS

Region	BMD[1] (g/cm²)	sBMD (mg/cm²)	Young-Adult[2,7] (%)	T-score	Age-Matched[3] (%)	Z-score	BMC (g)	Area (cm²)
Neck Left	0.919	840	89	-0.9	128	1.4	4.49	4.88
Neck Right	0.980	897	94	-0.4	136	1.9	4.89	4.99
Neck Mean	0.950	869	91	-0.6	132	1.7	4.69	4.94
Neck Diff.	0.061	57	6	0.4	8	0.4	0.41	0.11
Upper Neck Left	0.725	-	88	-0.8	126	1.3	1.74	2.40
Upper Neck Right	0.855	-	104	0.3	149	2.3	2.12	2.48
Upper Neck Mean	0.790	-	96	-0.3	138	1.8	1.93	2.44
Upper Neck Diff.	0.130	-	16	1.1	23	1.1	0.38	0.08
Lower Neck Left	1.107	-	-	-	-	-	2.75	2.48
Lower Neck Right	1.103	-	-	-	-	-	2.77	2.51
Lower Neck Mean	1.105	-	-	-	-	-	2.76	2.50
Lower Neck Diff.	0.004	-	-	-	-	-	0.02	0.03
Wards Left	0.725	-	80	-1.4	127	1.2	1.92	2.65
Wards Right	0.762	-	84	-1.1	133	1.5	2.11	2.77
Wards Mean	0.744	-	82	-1.3	130	1.3	2.01	2.71
Wards Diff.	0.037	-	4	0.3	6	0.3	0.19	0.12
Troch Left	0.716	-	84	-1.2	115	0.8	10.38	14.50
Troch Right	0.738	-	87	-1.0	118	1.0	10.30	13.97
Troch Mean	0.727	-	85	-1.1	116	0.9	10.34	14.24
Troch Diff.	0.022	-	3	0.2	4	0.2	0.08	0.54
Shaft Left	1.290	-	-	-	-	-	17.99	13.95
Shaft Right	1.286	-	-	-	-	-	17.60	13.69
Shaft Mean	1.288	-	-	-	-	-	17.79	13.82
Shaft Diff.	0.004	-	-	-	-	-	0.38	0.25
Total Left	0.986	934	98	-0.2	134	2.0	32.85	33.33
Total Right	1.004	952	100	0.0	137	2.1	32.80	32.65
Total Mean	0.995	943	99	-0.1	135	2.1	32.82	32.99
Total Diff.	0.019	18	2	0.1	3	0.1	0.05	0.68

1 - Statistically 68% of repeat scans fall within 1SD (± 0.010 g/cm² for DualFemur Total)
2 - USA (Combined NHANES (ages 20-30) / Lunar (ages 20-40)) Femur Reference Population (v113)
3 - Matched for Age, Weight (females 25-100 kg), Ethnic
7 - DualFemur Total T-score difference is 0.1. Asymmetry is None.
Filename: vqjemr6img.dfx

Fig. 6: Normal DEXA report of a patient, 80 years, female (Page 4).

Birth Date:	25-Jul-61 61.3 years	**Referring Physician:**			
Height / Weight:	156.0 cm 85.5 kg	**Measured:**	06-Dec-22	8:26:16 PM	(14.10)
Sex / Ethnic:	Female Asian	**Analyzed:**	09-Dec-22	1:04:55 PM	(14.10)

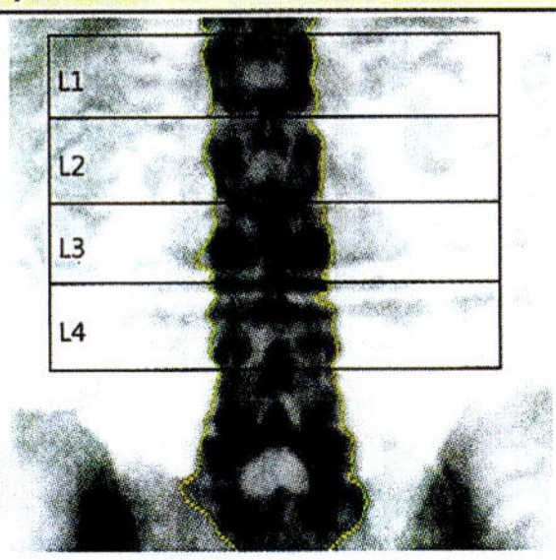

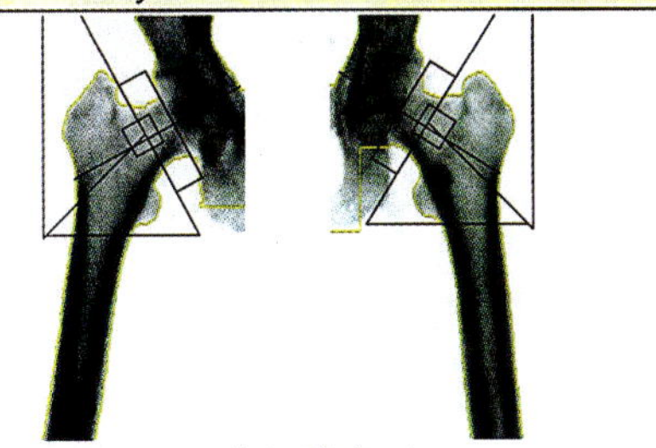

Image not for diagnosis

HAL chart results unavailable

Image not for diagnosis

(Right = 95.0 mm) (Left = 94.8 mm)

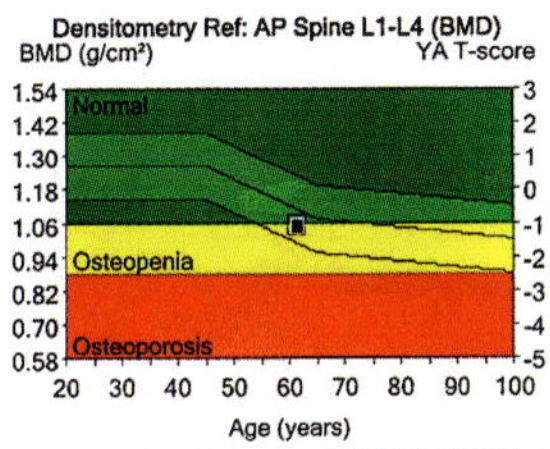

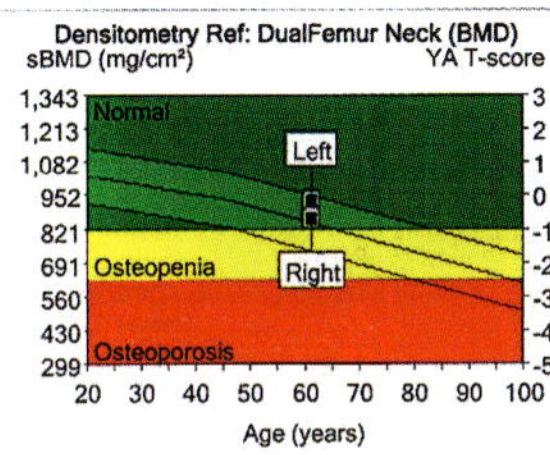

Region	sBMD (mg/cm²) [1]	Young-Adult T-score [2,7]	Age-Matched Z-score [3]	WHO Classification [11]
AP Spine L1-L4	-	-1.1	-0.5	Osteopenia
DualFemur Neck				
Left	933	-0.1	0.7	Normal
Right	862	-0.7	0.2	Normal
Mean	897	-0.4	0.4	Normal
Difference	71	0.5	0.5	-

1 - Statistically 68% of repeat scans fall within 1SD (± 0.010 g/cm² for AP Spine L1-L4); (± 13 mg/cm² for DualFemur Neck Right)
2 - USA (Combined NHANES (ages 20-30) / Lunar (ages 20-40)) AP Spine Reference Population (v113); USA (Combined NHANES (ages 20-30) / Lunar (ages 20-40)) Femur Reference Population (v113)
3 - AP Spine Matched for Age, Weight (females 25-100 kg), Ethnic; DualFemur Matched for Age, Weight (females 25-100 kg), Ethnic
7 - DualFemur Total T-score difference is 0.1. Asymmetry is None.
11 - World Health Organization - Definition of Osteoporosis and Osteopenia for Caucasian Women: Normal = T-score at or above -1.0 SD; Osteopenia = T-score between -1.0 and -2.5 SD; Osteoporosis = T-score at or below -2.5 SD; (WHO definitions only apply when a young healthy Caucasian Women reference database is used to determine T-scores.)

Fig. 7: DEXA report of a patient-2, 61F with osteopenia L spine, normal femurs (Page 1).

Patient ID:		**Birth Date:**	25-Jul-61	**Height:**	156.0 cm
Gender:	Female	**Exam Date:**	06-Dec-22	**Weight:**	85.5 kg
Indications:		**Fractures:**		**Treatments:**	

ASSESSMENT:

The BMD measured at AP Spine L1-L4 is 1.048 g/cm² with a T-score of -1.1. This patient is considered osteopenic according to World Health Organization (WHO) criteria. Bone density is between 10 and 25% below young normal. Fracture risk is moderate. Treatment is advised.

The BMD measured at Femur Neck Left is 1.018 g/cm² with a T-score of -0.1. Bone density is up to 10% below young normal. This patient is considered normal according to World Health Organization (WHO) criteria. Fracture risk is low.

The BMD measured at Femur Neck Right is 0.942 g/cm² with a T-score of -0.7. Bone density is up to 10% below young normal. This patient is considered normal according to World Health Organization (WHO) criteria. Fracture risk is low.

The BMD measured at Femur Total Left is 0.948 g/cm² with a T-score of -0.5. Bone density is up to 10% below young normal. This patient is considered normal according to World Health Organization (WHO) criteria. Fracture risk is low.

The BMD measured at Femur Total Right is 0.964 g/cm² with a T-score of -0.3. Bone density is up to 10% below young normal. This patient is considered normal according to World Health Organization (WHO) criteria. Fracture risk is low.

Site	Region	Measured Date	Measured Age	WHO Classification	Young Adult T-score	BMD
AP Spine	L1-L4	06-Dec-22	61.3	Osteopenia	-1.1	1.048 g/cm²
DualFemur	Neck Left	06-Dec-22	61.3	Normal	-0.1	1.018 g/cm²
DualFemur	Neck Right	06-Dec-22	61.3	Normal	-0.7	0.942 g/cm²
DualFemur	Total Left	06-Dec-22	61.3	Normal	-0.5	0.948 g/cm²
DualFemur	Total Right	06-Dec-22	61.3	Normal	-0.3	0.964 g/cm²

World Health Organization (WHO) criteria for post-menopausal, Caucasian Women:
Normal: T-score at or above -1 SD
Osteopenia: T-score between -1 and -2.5 SD
Osteoporosis: T-score at or below -2.5 SD

FOLLOW-UP:

People with diagnosed cases of osteoporosis or at high risk for fracture should have regular bone mineral density tests. For patients eligible for Medicare, routine testing is allowed once every 2 years. The testing frequency can be increased to one year for patients who have rapidly progressing disease, those who are receiving or discontinuing medical therapy to restore bone mass, or have additional risk factors.

Based on these results, a follow-up exam is recommended in December 2024

Fig. 8: DEXA Report of a patient-2, 61F with osteopenia L spine, normal femurs (Page 2).

Birth Date:	01-Jan-58 64.9 years	**Referring Physician:**			
Height / Weight:	142.0 cm 50.0 kg	**Measured:**	06-Dec-22	1:04:10 PM	(14.10)
Sex / Ethnic:	Female Asian	**Analyzed:**	09-Dec-22	12:56:46 PM	(14.10)

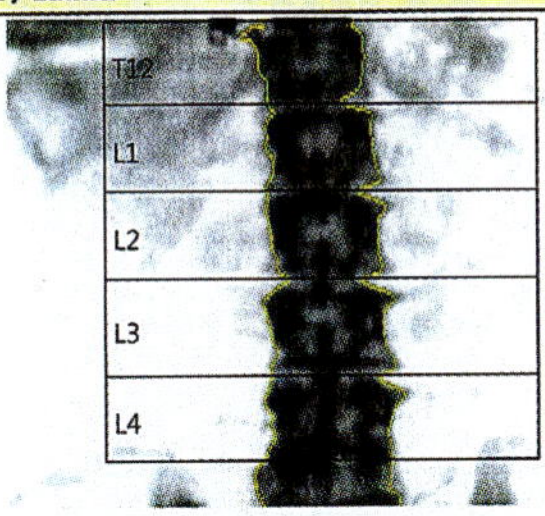

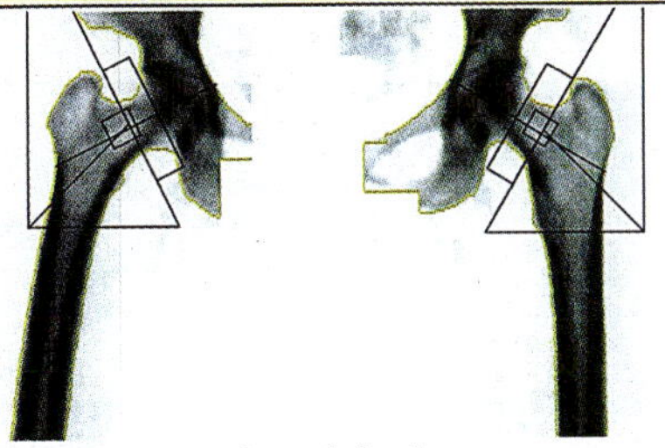

Image not for diagnosis

HAL chart results unavailable

Image not for diagnosis

(Right = 89.1 mm) (Left = 89.3 mm)

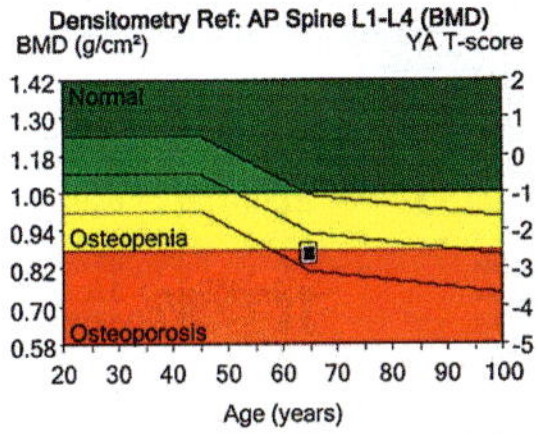

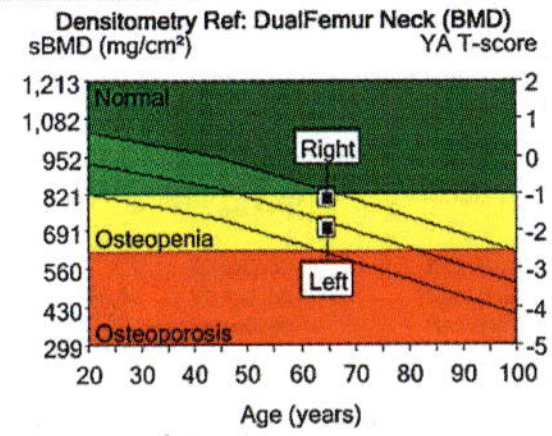

Region	sBMD[1] (mg/cm²)	Young-Adult[2,7] T-score	Age-Matched[3] Z-score	WHO Classification[11]
AP Spine L1-L4	-	-2.6	-0.6	Osteoporosis
DualFemur Neck				
Left	702	-1.9	-0.1	Osteopenia
Right	803	-1.1	0.6	Osteopenia
Mean	752	-1.5	0.2	Osteopenia
Difference	102	0.8	0.8	-

1 - Statistically 68% of repeat scans fall within 1SD (± 0.010 g/cm² for AP Spine L1-L4); (± 13 mg/cm² for DualFemur Neck Right)
2 - USA (Combined NHANES (ages 20-30) / Lunar (ages 20-40)) AP Spine Reference Population (v113); USA (Combined NHANES (ages 20-30) / Lunar (ages 20-40)) Femur Reference Population (v113)
3 - AP Spine Matched for Age, Weight (females 25-100 kg), Ethnic; DualFemur Matched for Age, Weight (females 25-100 kg), Ethnic
7 - DualFemur Total T-score difference is 1.6. Asymmetry is Significant.
11 - World Health Organization - Definition of Osteoporosis and Osteopenia for Caucasian Women: Normal = T-score at or above -1.0 SD; Osteopenia = T-score between -1.0 and -2.5 SD; Osteoporosis = T-score at or below -2.5 SD; (WHO definitions only apply when a young healthy Caucasian Women reference database is used to determine T-scores.)

Fig. 9: DEXA Report of a patient-3, 65F with osteoporosis L spine, osteopenia femurs (Page 1).

Patient ID:		**Birth Date:**	01-Jan-58	**Height:**	142.0 cm
Gender:	Female	**Exam Date:**	06-Dec-22	**Weight:**	50.0 kg
Indications:		**Fractures:**		**Treatments:**	

ASSESSMENT:

The BMD measured at AP Spine L1-L4 is 0.865 g/cm² with a T-score of -2.6. This patient is considered osteoporotic according to World Health Organization (WHO) criteria. Fracture risk is high. Pharmacological treatment, if not already prescribed, should be started. A follow up bone density test is recommended in one year to monitor response to therapy.

The BMD measured at Femur Neck Left is 0.772 g/cm² with a T-score of -1.9. This patient is considered osteopenic according to World Health Organization (WHO) criteria. Bone density is between 10 and 25% below young normal. Fracture risk is moderate. Treatment is advised.

The BMD measured at Femur Neck Right is 0.880 g/cm² with a T-score of -1.1. This patient is considered osteopenic according to World Health Organization (WHO) criteria. Bone density is between 10 and 25% below young normal. Fracture risk is moderate. Treatment is advised.

The BMD measured at Femur Total Left is 0.736 g/cm² with a T-score of -2.2. This patient is considered osteopenic according to World Health Organization (WHO) criteria. Bone density is between 10 and 25% below young normal. Fracture risk is moderate. Treatment is advised.

The BMD measured at Femur Total Right is 0.937 g/cm² with a T-score of -0.6. Bone density is up to 10% below young normal. This patient is considered normal according to World Health Organization (WHO) criteria. Fracture risk is low.

Site	Region	Measured Date	Measured Age	WHO Classification	Young Adult T-score	BMD
AP Spine	L1-L4	06-Dec-22	64.9	Osteoporosis	-2.6	0.865 g/cm²
DualFemur	Neck Left	06-Dec-22	64.9	Osteopenia	-1.9	0.772 g/cm²
DualFemur	Neck Right	06-Dec-22	64.9	Osteopenia	-1.1	0.880 g/cm²
DualFemur	Total Left	06-Dec-22	64.9	Osteopenia	-2.2	0.736 g/cm²
DualFemur	Total Right	06-Dec-22	64.9	Normal	-0.6	0.937 g/cm²

World Health Organization (WHO) criteria for post-menopausal, Caucasian Women:
Normal: T-score at or above -1 SD
Osteopenia: T-score between -1 and -2.5 SD
Osteoporosis: T-score at or below -2.5 SD

FOLLOW-UP:

People with diagnosed cases of osteoporosis or at high risk for fracture should have regular bone mineral density tests. For patients eligible for Medicare, routine testing is allowed once every 2 years. The testing frequency can be increased to one year for patients who have rapidly progressing disease, those who are receiving or discontinuing medical therapy to restore bone mass, or have additional risk factors.

Based on these results, a follow-up exam is recommended in December 2023

Fig. 10: DEXA report of a patient-3, 65F with osteoporosis L spine, osteopenia femurs (Page 2).

TAKE-HOME POINTS

- DEXA is quick, easy to perform and non-invasive.
- DEXA does not require any sedation or anesthesia.
- DEXA provides precise information about fracture risk.
- DEXA involves very little radiation exposure.
- DEXA is an appropriate screening test and is able to detect disease (osteoporosis or osteopenia) at a stage when treatment (medication or lifestyle modification) can effectively reduce the serious consequences such as fracture.
- DEXA is safe, widely available and affordable.

Balancing Exercises for Fall and Fracture Prevention in Osteoporosis

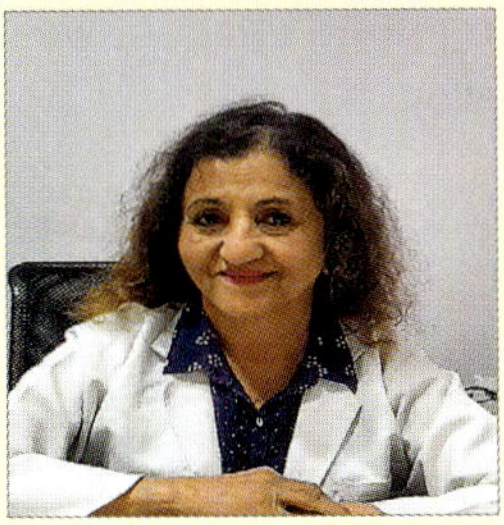

Compiler
Dr Maninder Ahuja

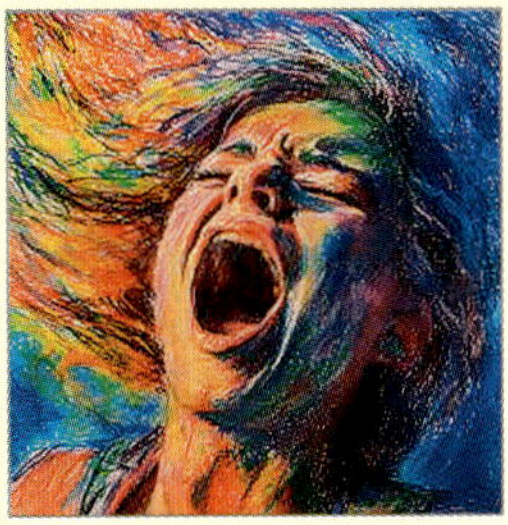

Fractures are painful

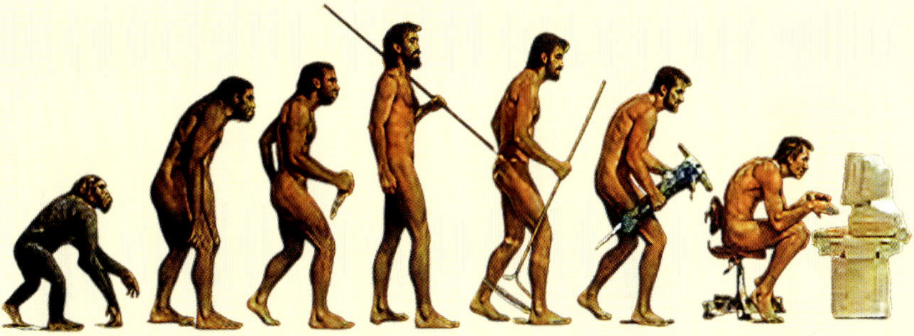

Aging is not inevitable inactivity or wrong type of activity is going to be harmful

One in three women >55 years of age suffer from Osteoporosis! Osteoporosis is silent but fractures are not silent they are painful and cause loss of life and long physical impairment and huge expenditure.

How body keeps balance for preventing falls?

In *preventing falls* there are two basic types of balance:

1. *Static balance* gives the ability to stand up without falling over,
2. *Dynamic balance* allows to anticipate and react to changes as we move.

Four systems in our body work together to help stay balanced:

1. The central nervous system coordinates movements by sending motor signals to the eyes and muscles
2. The vestibular system of the inner ear sends messages to the brain about the position and movements of your head in relation to the ground
3. Vision helps balance by showing where bodies are in relation to other objects
4. Position-sensing nerves—called proprioceptors—embedded in muscles, tendons and joints throughout body help move around without stumbling or bumping into things.

Exercises to Prevent Falls and Fractures

As we age, we are at risk of falling or tripping. This can result in broken bones or even more serious injuries because of compound effect of weak bones, weak muscles, poor hearing, vision, and reflexes.

Exercising can help prevent falls because it can:

- Make muscles stronger and more flexible
- Improve balance
- Increase how long you can be active or maintain balance
- All adult women should engage in 150 minutes per week of moderate to vigorous aerobic activity exercise and
- Three days resistance training of all muscles of body should be added.

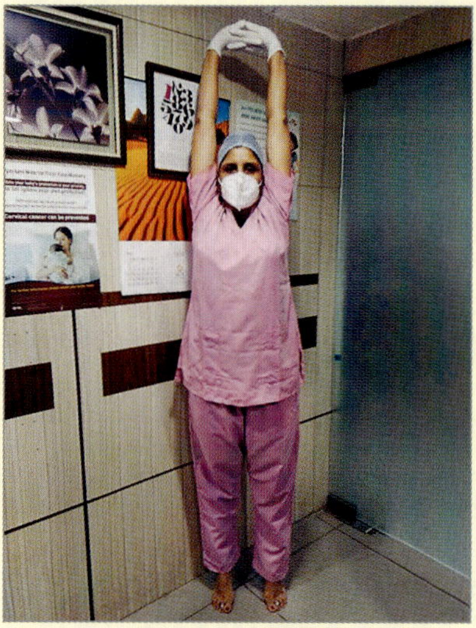

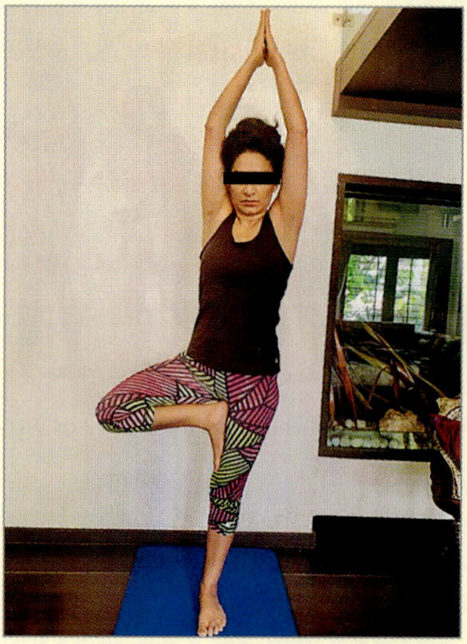

Quadriceps stretch

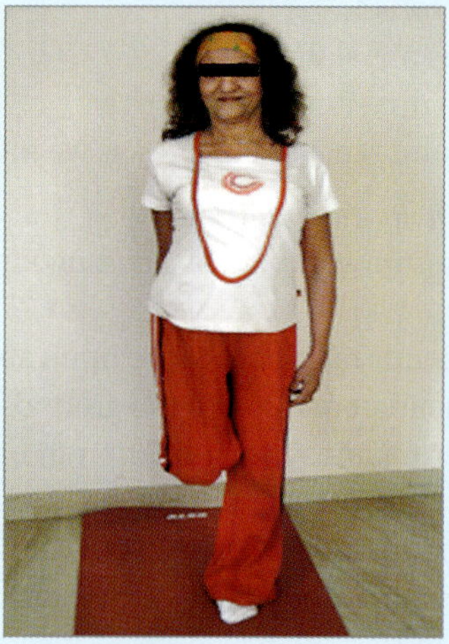

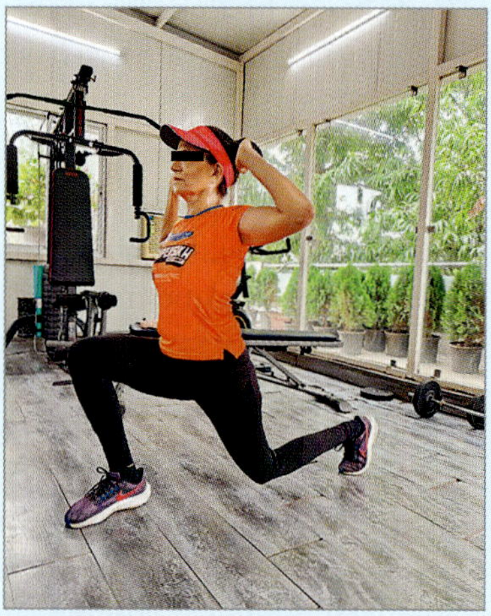

Any time. Any where!

First Step Right Posture

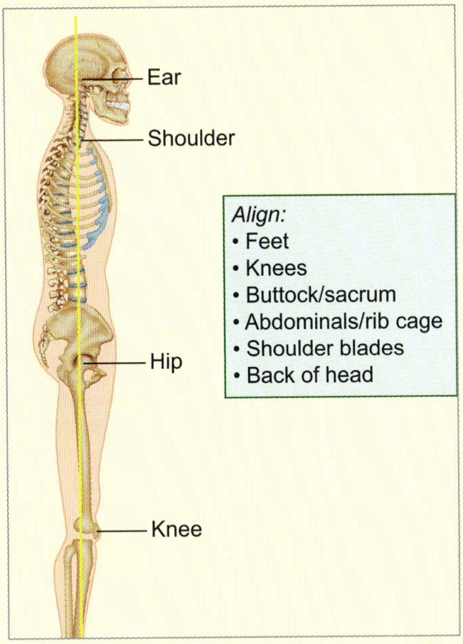

Don't bend spine!

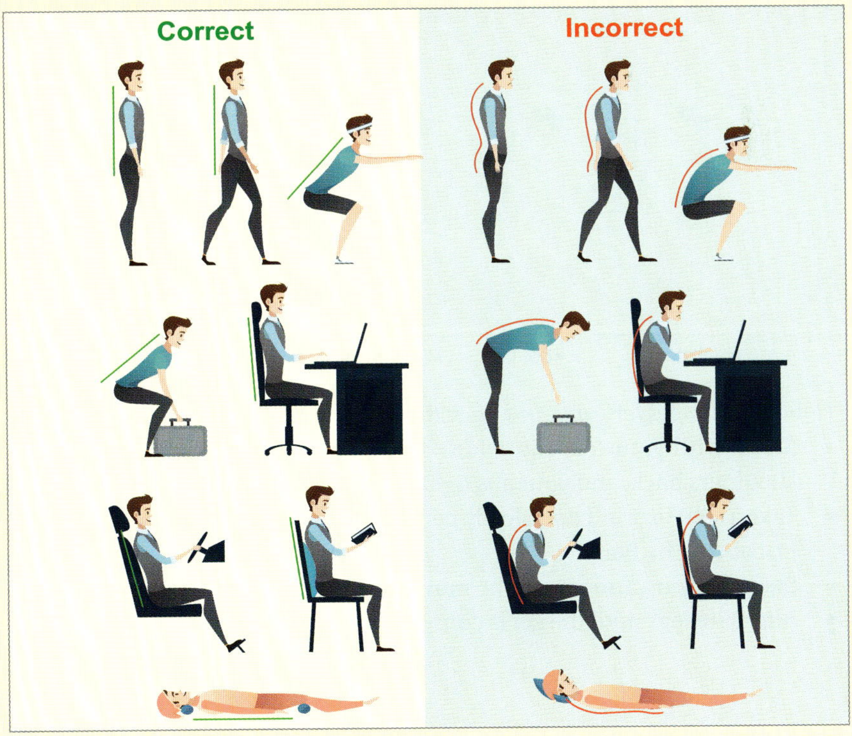

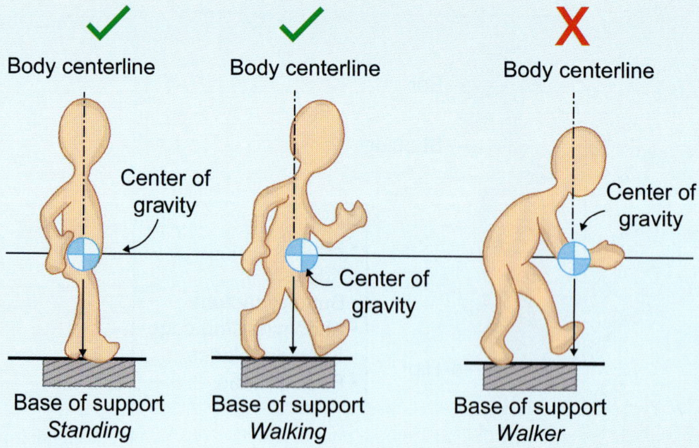

Steps of balance:

- Alignment of body
- Standing tall
- Standing on toes
- Standing on one foot –25 seconds
- Standing on one foot eyes closed >6 seconds
- Walking properly
- Take support of chair while learning

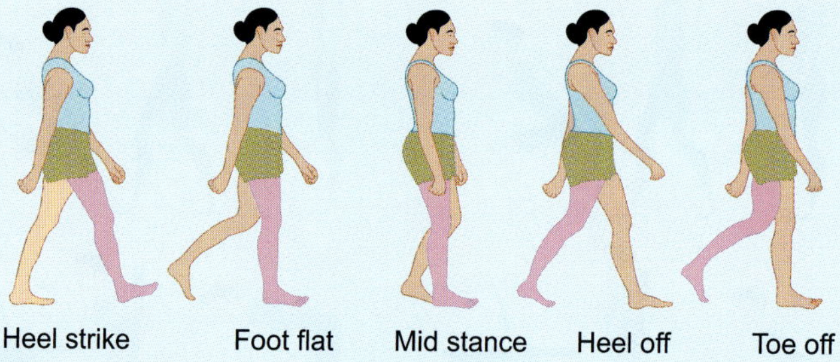

How to do lunges for front and back thigh:

- Stand with your feet hip-width apart, keep your back straight, your shoulders back, and your abs tight.
- Take a step forward and slowly bend both knees, until your back knee is just above the floor.
- Stand back up and repeat the movement.
- Alternate legs until the set is complete.

Rock Step-balance and Move

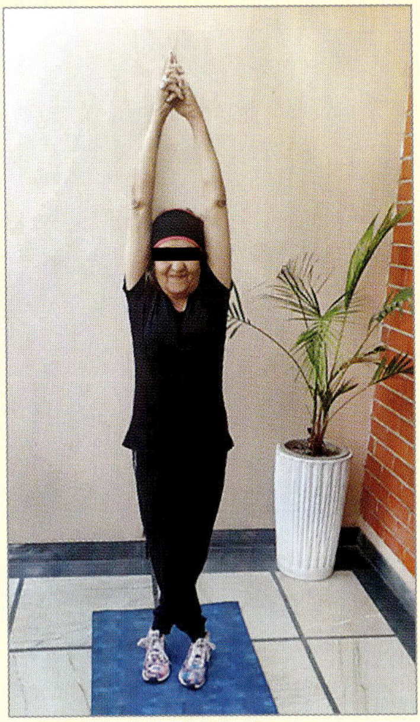 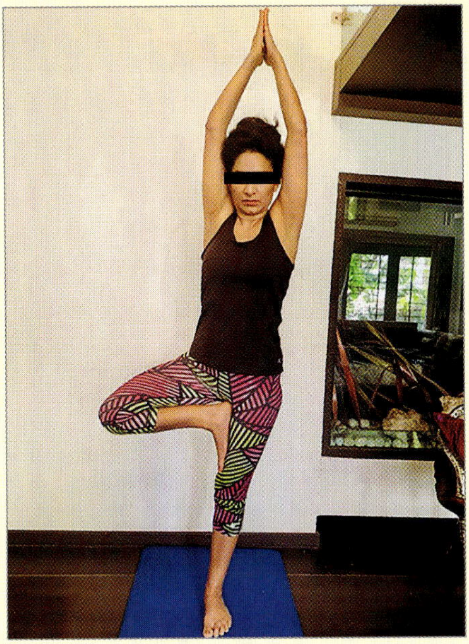

Static Exercise

Feet Together

Stand with your feet touching or as close together as you feel comfortable. Maintain a tall upright posture and hold this position for 10–60 seconds as tolerated.

Semi-Tandem Stand

Stand with the toes of one foot should be touching the arch of the other. Maintain a tall upright posture and hold this position for 10–60 seconds as tolerated. Repeat on the other side.

Tandem Stand

Stand with one front directly in front of the other, the toes of one foot touching the heel of the other. Stand as tall and still as you are able to for 10–60 seconds. Repeat with the other leg.

Single Leg Stand

Stand on one leg while maintaining a tall, upright position. Begin with 10 second hold on each leg and gradually build your way up to 60 seconds per leg.

Tandem Stand

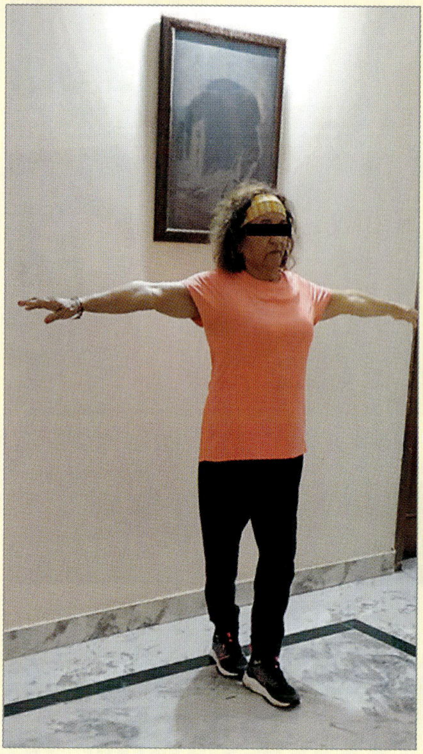

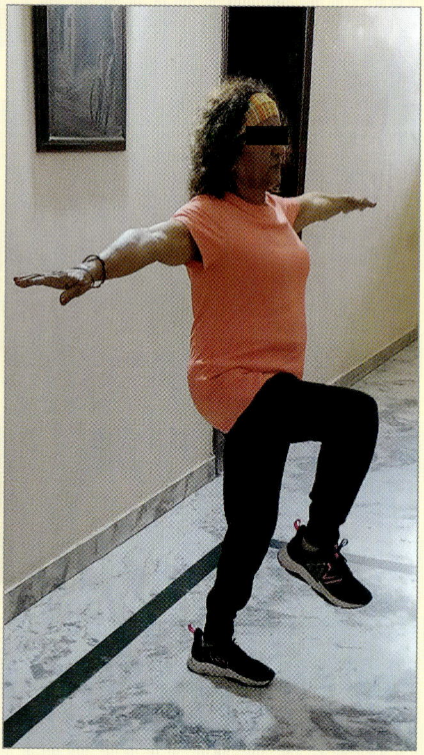

Stand up straight, feet hip-width apart and weight distributed evenly on both feet. Put your arms at your sides and brace your abdominal muscles.

Place your left foot directly in front of your right foot, heel to toe, and squeeze your inner thighs together. Lift your arms out to your sides at shoulder level to help you balance. Hold. Return to the starting position, then repeat with your right foot in front. This completes one rep.

Balance by Walking in a Pattern –Tandem Walk

- Heel to toe

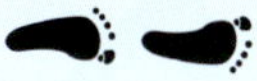

- *Step aerobics:* Two narrow steps, then two wide steps

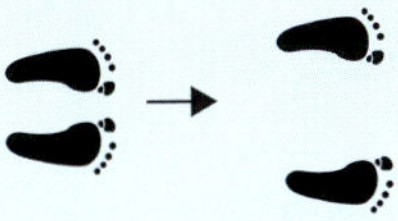

- Sideways or grapevine

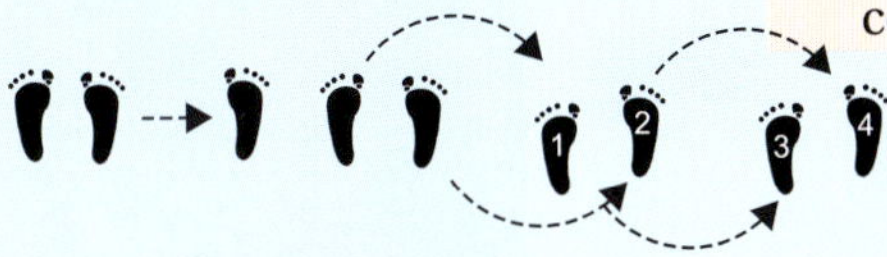

Try walking in an unusual pattern to challenge your balance.

Walk with this pattern for ________.

Here are some other ones you can try:

- Step over cones or cups
- Walk in a figure 8
- Walk forward or backward, and count forward by 6s
- Walk forward or backward, and count backward by 6s

Strengthen Muscles of Legs and Back

Squats with the support of a wall

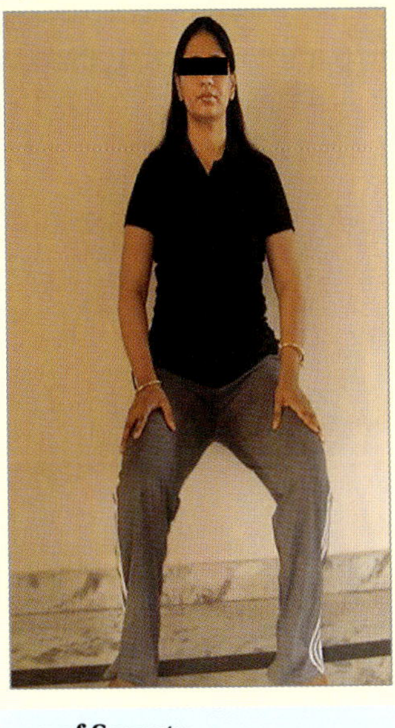

Lunges with weights

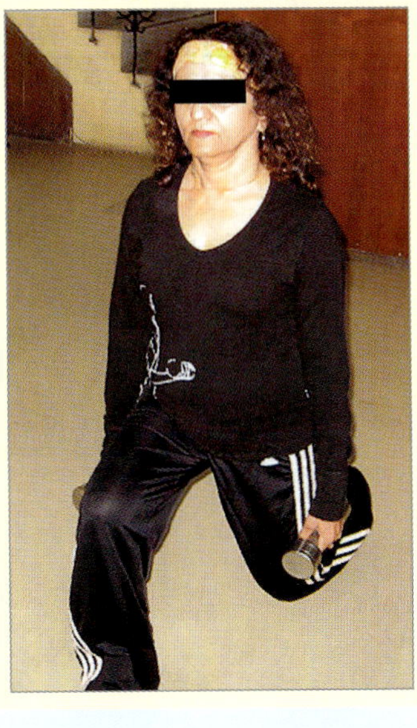

Steps of Squats

1. Step 1: Stand straight with feet hip-width apart. ...
2. Step 2: Engage your core muscles. ...
3. Step 3: Lower down, as if sitting in an invisible chair. ...
4. Step 4: Lift back up to standing position. ...
5. Step 5: Repeat for 10 to 15 reps, for three sets.

Lunges without weight

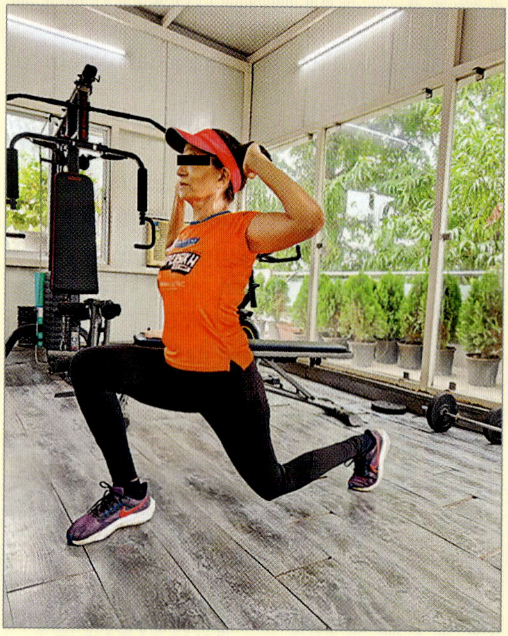

Aerobic cycling

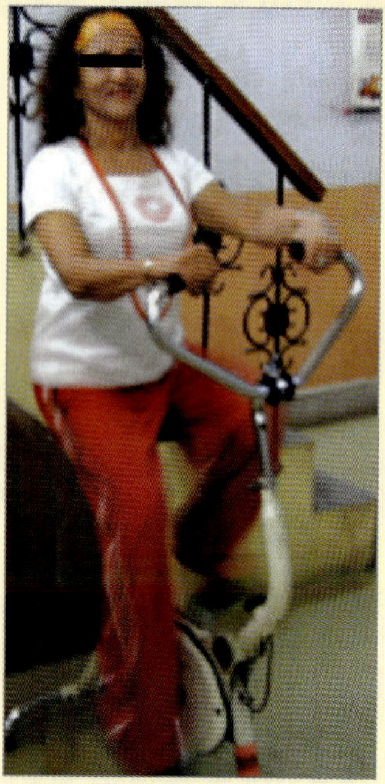

Precautions in Homes

Good lighting at night, no clutter, handrails in bathrooms, stools for taking bath, do not lock bathroom.

Hip Hinges to Prevent Spine Flexion
Spine fractures

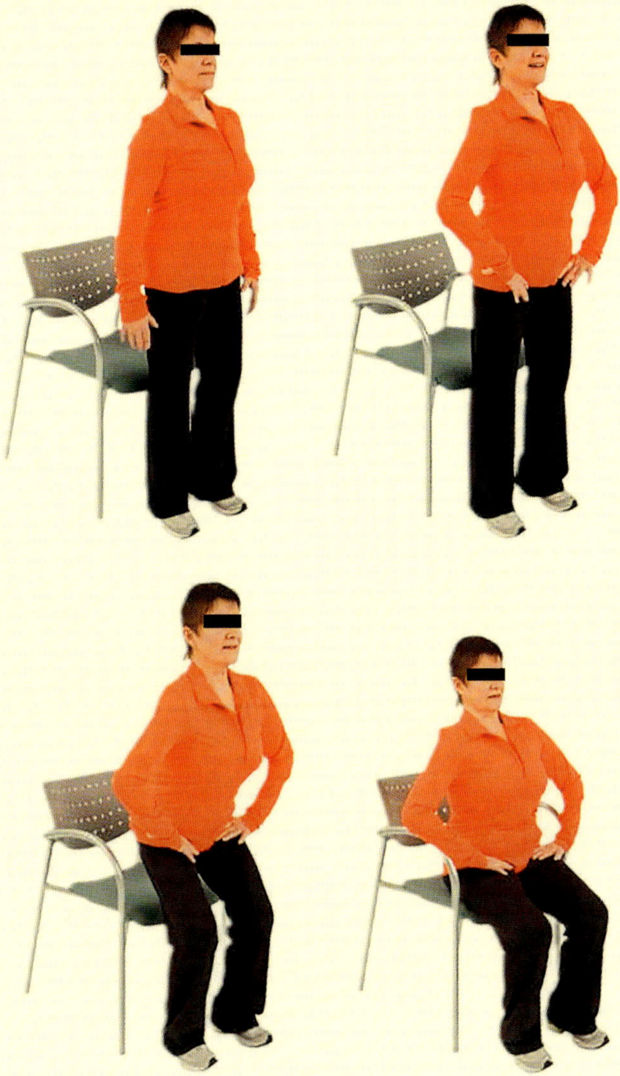

1. Start with standing with good postural alignment
2. Place hands in the creases of your hips
3. Bend at the hips over your hands sticking your bottom out slightly and keeping back straight alignment
4. Lower yourself gently onto chair keeping this alignment

When ever picking. Objects from floor don't bend your spine, bend over knees. Rotate feet and not your spine when turning.